ANN ANTOGNOLI

A Heart so Wide

HOPE LIVES WHEN LOVE LISTENS

This book is a work of fiction. The characters, incidents, and dialogue are products of the author's imagination and are not to be construed as real.

First Printing 2018

Printed by Create Space. Charleston, SC

Available from Amazon.com and other book stores

Ann Antognoli, Publisher

ISBN: 978-0-9960241-3-6 (for print version)
ISBN: 978-0-9960241-2-9 (for kindle version)

End child abuse.
Listen when they tell you.

The world stands out on either side
No wider than the heart is wide;
Above the world is stretched the sky,
No higher than the soul is high.
The heart can push the sea and land
Farther away on either hand;
The soul can split the sky in two,
And let the face of God shine through.
But East and West will pinch the heart
That cannot keep them pushed apart;
And he whose soul is flat—the sky
Will cave in on him by and by.

Edna St. Vincent Millay, from the poem "Renascence"

Chapter One

SAMANTHA KIND HAD A LOT TO SAY ABOUT A WORLD THAT remained silent while adults abused children. In her mind, people didn't care. If they did, Jenna Rossi, marred by her own dance with depravity, wouldn't be the only one who possessed a heart so wide and a touch of guilt to keep listening to her, to keep fighting for her.

"Why didn't anyone help me?" Sam asked, her bottle clinking on an empty glass. "If only one person would've helped me. The whole neighborhood had to know what he was doing to me, Jen."

Growing up in her quiet suburban neighborhood, Jenna Rossi and her friends never had an inkling of Sam's plight. It wasn't until the day Sam shot and killed her father, seconds after she claimed her father murdered her mother, that Sam began to reveal the saga of her torturous childhood to anyone who would listen. Each time Sam told the tale, she unearthed a new, dark detail reminding Jenna that there's evil in the world strong enough to cloud the light of hope we lend each other.

Held captive by Sam's tirade on speaker phone, Jenna sat in her car, ready to bolt at the first break in a caravan of busses leaving the school parking lot. Her hand blindly reached over and rummaged through her bright, red purse propped up on the passenger's seat. Grabbing a tube of lipstick, she told Sam, "They've been dead all these years. Stop giving the monsters power over you."

Sam pounded her head against a wall and garbled, "Ican'tstop. I hear 'em. Over and over and over. They're draggin' me under, Jen. Likea big ol' sinkin' ship." She took in three deep breaths, paused, and let out a loud wail. "Whyyy? What kinda father," she sucked in her breath, held it for a second, and whispered, "rapes a baby?" Her voice shook when she cried, "Myyy ooown faaather." Sniffling for several seconds, her voice turned cold and detached when she said, "My mother told me, 'That's what men do.'"

Jenna glanced at her watch, ran lipstick over her lips, and smacked them together. Just enough time to make my hair appointment, she thought.

"Funny you compare yourself to a sinking ship, Sam. When Josh and I complained, my grandfather would always tell us, 'Keep the water out of the ship.' Focus on the positives, girlfriend. Let's plan some fun for my visit in a few days."

"You want me to focus better?" She took another drink. "All ly mife . . . I mean my life, I've stumbled 'round like a blind man, and all you can say is, 'Focus better'?"

Jenna dabbed her lips one more time, smacked them together, and tossed the tube into her purse.

Annoyed by the distraction, Sam asked, "What's that noise?"

"I'm evening out my lipstick is all."

"That makes me feel so special. I'm, I'msinking. I'm drowning and . . ." a soft burp escaped her, "and yer . . . You onlycare 'bout dolling yourselfup?"

"Stop picking on me, Sam. I'm multi-tasking."

"Whocaresanyway?" she mumbled, words that measured the futility of her state of being. "People in that whole neighborhood, maybe the whole goddamn world, were puttin' makeup on their ugly faces. All the while my screwedup dad . . . Almost every night, dy mad . . . I mean my dad hurt me." In between garbling other insinuations, she said, "Goahead, put makeup on." Letting loose a louder burp, she mumbled, "Makeup can't crover up . . . won't cover up the truth."

After a longer than usual silence, Jenna asked, "You still there?"

"Course I'm here. Where'm I gonnago?" Sam shattered the moments of silence with a sudden attack, screaming, "Why didn't anyone help me?"

Lurching forward, Jenna palmed her chest and said, "Gosh, Sam! You almost sent me through the windshield."

"Almost doesn't count," she said, pouting.

Plagued by her friend's phone calls that moved from childish day dreams to bitter reality in seconds, Jenna grew accustomed to Sam's memories tumbling around in her head and pouring out in a flurry of confusion. Her drunken ramblings told the tale of an only child raised in a crucible of isolation and loneliness until kindergarten lent her some relief. Sam managed to maneuver around the unrealistic expectations of a sadomasochistic mother and father until their deaths loosened their grip on her. Early on, she learned to dull her senses with less judgmental friends, Jack Daniels one day and Johnnie Walker the next, until one by one, her few childhood friends withered and dropped away, poisoned by frequent revelations of her obscene family history.

"Listening to you and putting on lipstick at the same time is one of the easier functions in life," Jenna told Sam. "If I plopped in a chair and just listened every time you held me captive, my legs would atrophy."

Hiccups interrupted Sam's laughter. Pausing to allow a louder burp to escape, she asked, "'Member the last time I threatened to kill myself? You wouldn't let me. You wouldn't hangup 'til I got tired. I'm sooo tired, Jen." Her voice turned sweet. "You're my only friend. I love you to the moon and back. Love you as deep . . . as deep as the 'Cific Ocean. As wide as—"

"I get it, Sam, but what's a 'Cific Ocean?"

"Pacific Ocean, okay?" Sam yelled. "Don't criticize someone givin' you a compliment."

"Sounds like you have a touch of post dramatic stress syndrome going on, Samantha."

"I do! No, really, Jenna. My analyst said I have stress from all the childhood trauma. You think I like bein' this way? They stole my life. They picked and picked and picked. Like I was a scab . . . a scab on a cut."

As her eyes followed the busses passing in her rearview mirror, Jenna said, "I told you how my mother reported your dad to Child Protective Services. You moved before the authorities could haul his ass to court."

"Oooh yeaaah. My dad did his job so good; they promoted the bastard." Her glass clinked against the bottle as she poured another drink. "Some people fly high in the sky; some people get jacked in the crack." Gulping more whiskey, she began slurring a song. "HereIam, Lord, hight ere, trapped in a little ol' crack in this biguglyworld." Fearing retaliation from the silent shadows of her brutal past, she whispered, "Does God have any idea how stinky, dark, and really scary it is in this cesspool He created?" After another quick drink, she said more lucidly, as though it were a fresh insight, "Mothers and fathers should protect their babies. Babies aren't supposed to cater to their crazy, drunken parents."

Wanton memories induced agonizing groans as she shrank from imaginings of ghosts that had the power to rise from their graves and have their way with her all over again.

The day after Sam's eighteenth birthday, newspapers recorded the heinous account of her father in a drunken rage murdering her mother, and Sam shooting her father after a struggle because she feared for her own life. Their deaths promised relief, but respite was short-lived. Deep-seated distortions about life took hold before Sam learned to walk and talk and metastasized throughout her teen years. Distrust of people, particularly fear of men, was branded in her psyche by the time her parents forgot to celebrate her fifth birthday.

Separated from her tormentors by six feet of earth freed her to tell her story to childhood friends scattered on college campuses throughout the country. At first, willing to endure hours of soliloquies filled with gruesome revelations, Sam's friends wearied when she described heinous acts that she had told them many times before. When they compared notes and confided in their parents, the most arduous hearts debated whether the tales Sam told were real or delusions of a sick mind. What remained consistent in her tales, between comical snorts and gut-wrenching groans, were Sam's questions, "Why didn't anyone help me? Why didn't anyone love me?"

Jenna, a high school English teacher, trained to recognize child abuse, never blamed Sam for asking the wholly reasonable questions. As far as she was concerned, the physical and emotional damage Sam's parents inflicted on her defied credulity. More incredulous was her mother's compliance with her husband's violent masculinity toward her daughter.

At least once a week Sam reminded Jenna of the time a pair of volunteers from the Child Protective Services visited their elementary school to entertain the class with a puppet show focusing on *stranger danger*, a child's age-appropriate guide to teach the difference between good touches and bad touches. Confused by information that conflicted with her life experiences, Sam naively wondered if her mother was aware that her father's brutality toward them both was wrong. Eager to share the news with her mother, she pushed open the back door and found her mother leaning against the kitchen counter sipping on a glass of vodka. Hesitating for an instant, Sam blurted out, "Did you know we could tell people not to touch our private parts if we want? Miss Ryan said—"

Eyes bulging, her mother pointed at Sam and warned in a hissing voice, "Don't you ever talk about who touches yer private parts to anyone." Her voice shaking, she asked, "You didn't blab, did you?"

Wagging her head hard, Sam said, "I didn't tell! Honest I didn't!"

Well on her way to intoxication, her mother gulped her drink and said snarling, "If you would've stopped cryin' . . . If you would've kept the house cleaner, he would've left us alone."

"But one time you told me he started bothering me when I was a baby. Babies don't know how to—"

Pouring another drink, her mother yelled, "Smart ones do!" Glaring at Sam, she said, "That teacher probably opens her legs as much as she opens her mouth. Men are all the same. Just give 'em what they want." Her hot eyes pierced Sam. "I can't count how many times he beat me 'cause you wouldn't shut that screechin' mouth." She turned to wipe the already immaculate counter. Her hands visibly shaking, she lined up the salt and pepper shakers, and said, "You got what you deserved." Wringing the dishcloth, she gritted her teeth, and said, "I wanted to smother you so many times." She spun around, shot Sam a cold, matter of fact stare, and said, "But then he would've been all over me."

Deaf to her mother's death wish for her, Sam pleaded, "Why can't we run away, Mom? Miss Ryan said they let people like us stay at the—"

A wild look crossed her mother's face. Loud and shrill, she spewed angry words. "Screw Miss Ryan, and screw you, you moron! What does that woman know about people like us?" She lunged at Sam, grabbed her mouth, and dug her long, manicured nails into Sam's cheeks. "I should rip out yer tongue right now! If you go around tellin' anyone what you think I said or what you think your dad does to you, they'll drop you in a foster home so fast, and then you'll see who all touches yer private parts." Sam felt her mother's hot breath reeking with alcohol on her face as her mother's teeth nipped her cheek. With a vicious whisper, she told Sam, "You'll have more fingerprints on yer body than the FBI has in its files." She wiped her mouth with a paper towel, discarded it, and carefully matched up the ends of the dish towel, folded it perfectly, and gently patted it on the counter. Filling her glass to the rim, she turned to make her way to the den, and warned, "Stay outta my sight."

On the heels of her mother, Sam fought back hot tears, and said, "Last week you told me how sorry you were because I was only a baby when he first made me . . . made me . . ." Sam burst into sobs and sputtered, "He hurts me, Mom. Miss Ryan said . . . She said we should keep telling 'til—"

Her mother turned, swung her closed fist at Sam, and landed a hard blow on the right side of her head. Sam dropped to the floor, her head reeling.

Unleashing a torrid, verbal assault, her mother yelled, "Yer more worthless than the shit I flushed down the toilet this morning. Whaaa . . . whaaa . . . whaaa," she mocked. "He threw a can of beer at me because you wouldn't stop bawlin." Palming her chest, she said, "He knocked me to the floor and forced me to clean it up." Glaring, she asked, "You have any idea what it feels like to be his slave?"

Sam pounded the floor with her clenched fists. "Why don't you give me away? Jenna's mom wishes she had another little girl. I wanna live with them."

Her mother let out a loud cackle. "Dream on, ya little wart. Like those people really want someone as pathetic and stupid as you trollin' 'round their prissy house. All's yer good for is keepin' this house clean and keepin' yer crazy father away from me." Mocking Sam, she said, "Yer goin' nowhere with no one, so get used to it."

Sam stood, glared at her mother, and said, "Next time Miss Ryan asks me how I bruised my legs, I'm tellin' the tru—"

In an instant, Sam's mother lunged at her, grabbed a handful of her hair, and yanked hard. Pressing Sam's face into the floor, she threatened, "I'll lock you in the basement until you rot with the rats if you breathe one word of our business." She yanked Sam's head up and shoved her face into Sam's face. Through clenched teeth, she said, "Our business," she twisted Sam's hair tighter, "is our business." Sam's long, agonizing wails shook the walls. Begging her mother to stop hurting her, she cried, "I won't tell! I won't; I won't."

Seeing red, her mother slammed Sam's head onto the floor once more, stood, and gave her a swift kick in the side. With a sinister whisper, she warned, "Don't let your dad catch wind of all yer private parts and woman shelter talk. Not a word!" she hissed. "He'll take a shotgun to both of us."

Sprawled on the floor, Sam whimpered like a wounded animal until her mother's demonic scream sent a jolt through her. "Get up, you half-wit! Clean this place up! Don't give him anything to complain about." Before she walked away, she looked down at the battered heap and casually said, "Quit actin' like yer the martyr of the century."

From that moment until she buried her parents, Sam bore her abuse in silence.

"Yer mom would've killed to protect you, Jen. My mother used me." A short silence passed before she asked, "Whocaresanyway?"

Jenna sympathized saying, "They were sick, Sam. All your mother knew was fear and abuse. The liquor didn't help, and it sure isn't helping you."

Sam garbled the standard alcoholic's excuse: "I canstop anytime. AnytimeIwant, Jen. Some people use," a hiccup escaped her, "pills; I use whiskey for medicinalpurposes."

"Your doctor can't prescribe useful meds if you're always bombed out of your mind, Sam."

Adept at disregarding Jenna's reprimands, she said, as though it were a first-time revelation, "Did I ever tell you my father invited his friends over when my mom . . . My mother loved playing Bingo.

Ohhh, yeaaah." She let loose a sarcastic laugh and said, "I bet some nights I made more money than she did. Sometimes he'd flick a quarter at me. That's how much I'm worth. Twenty-five pennies." After a short pause she asked, "Whocaresanyway?"

Seizing an opening in the traffic, Jenna began easing out of the parking space when a loud, angry voice shouted, "Don't do this to me!"

She slammed the brake and darted her eyes to the car parked to the right of her. Mike Gaone sat glaring with such intensity that she expected any second for his steering wheel to melt in his hands.

Unleashing a second outburst, he bellowed, "I need help right now, Dad!" as Sam whined, "Why won't you come see me, Jen? I need help with—"

Jenna interrupted Sam and said, "I have to go. One of my students has a problem."

Miffed, Sam complained, "If you wanna be a problem solver, come here and help me clean this pigsty." Protesting, she asked, "Know what it feels like to be infested with bugs crawlin' all over the place? A fly's been buzzin' 'round my kitchen for days makin' me lose what's left of my mind. More crap's 'round here than a manure farm. I haven't eaten a hot meal in weeks, and I swear . . . I know someone stole . . . They lifted my credit card when I stopped at that pizza shop the other day. They're probably throwin' a block party with a buffet of drugs, compliments of yours truly." Her anger subsided into sniffles that resembled a sump pump working beyond its capacity.

"Sam, I pick up every time you call. I don't know whose house you're describing, but it sure isn't the one you live in. Take a good look around you, girlfriend. Your house is more sterile than a Johns Hopkins operating room seconds before pediatric neurosurgery. The fumes from all that bleach you use are enough to induce a coma. You don't eat because cooking and eating make crumbs and that dirties your kitchen." Exasperated, she asked, "And how many more times do I have to tell you that no one stole your credit card? The last time you lost it, I was looking for frozen waffles and found it stuffed in a brown paper bag tucked in your freezer. For God's sake, let me see what this kid needs. He's right in front of me; you're over an hour away. I promise I'll call back tonight."

Seeping sarcasm, Sam said, "Thanks for nothin', friend."

The familiar, hard click jabbed Jenna with guilt as she turned to Mike and called out, "What's the problem, kiddo?"

Slamming the steering wheel with his free hand, he said, "My car died!" Snapping his eyes shut, he added, "Coach Shaffer wants us to meet some football scouts in an hour." Dramatically holding the phone up in front of his face, his voice oozed disdain saying, "But my father refuses to help me because he doesn't want to offend some fat-cat client who won't stop talking!"

Irked by his son's over-simplification of the attention he afforded his client who promised to yield substantial profit to his company, Stephen Gaone warned, "Mouth off one more time, Mike, and you'll be landing on the moon without a lunar module." His heavy exhale signaled mounting impatience. "Stop whining and call Nonna or Uncle Phil."

"I tried that, Dad. No one answers!" Leveling a grievance, he added, "It's like nobody cares if I exist."

Jenna waved Mike into her car and said, "I'll take you to where you need to be."

Mike's face reddened, but he breathed easier. Sitting in her passenger seat, Mike asked his dad, "Are you still there?"

"Not for long."

"My English teacher offered to drop me off." Thinking of the awkwardness of having her in the house while he showered and changed, he told his father, "I guess I'll wear what I have on and be a little early."

Rolling her eyes, she held out her hand, and said, "Let me talk to your father." Clearing her throat, she said, "Mr. Gaone, this is Jenna Rossi. I'll take Mike home, wait in the car while he cleans up, then I'll drive him to the banquet center." Winking at Mike, she said, "Now both Gaone men can dazzle tonight."

Steve's voice carried appreciation saying, "Thanks for doing some dazzling yourself. One more word from that kid, I was going to—"

"Stop right there, Mr. Gaone. The law mandates that teachers need to report suspected child abuse."

Caught off guard for a moment, he said, "Let me modify. I owe you dinner."

"A can of ginger ale will even the score. Besides," she said with levity, "some wealthy client might want to talk; you'll stand me up, and I'd starve."

"Ouch! That infant in your car painted a false impression of his devoted dad."

"I bet he did. I imagine some of your clients are like some of my parents at *Meet the Teacher Night*. When ten o'clock rolls around, all I crave is to kick off my heels and plop on the couch, but moms and dads can't resist singing the praises of their progeny 'til the rooster crows."

"I'm a firm believer that there's a thread of good in every crisis. It took Mike's car dying for me finally to find someone who understands what it's like to be held hostage by people who bolster one's livelihood." Sounding rushed, he said, "Be on the lookout for a case of ginger ale."

Mike showered, dressed, and jumped into Jenna's car fifteen minutes before the start of the banquet. He caught the tail end of a car phone conversation Jenna was having with her beautician.

"Sorry, Jen. Right now, I'm swamped. Unless you're Cinderella going to the ball, the soonest I can reschedule you is next Saturday at one."

He detected disappointment in Jenna's voice when she said, "Okay, pen me in. I apologize for the no-show."

She entered the new date into her phone and asked, "To what banquet center am I taking you, young man?"

"The one two blocks from the police station."

Uneasy about interfering with her personal life, Mike glanced at her sideways and asked, "I screwed up your hair appointment, didn't I?"

Waving her hand, she said, "I've gone longer between cuts."

Her laid-back tone put him at ease. Dialing down some of the negativity he spun about his father, he said, "Just so you know, my dad's not that bad." He shot her a crooked grin. "Man, I really ticked him off. He doesn't get that mad at anyone."

Shooting him a quick glance, she said, "You were quite the fire-breathing dragon yourself, kiddo."

He raised his eyebrows and said, "Guaranteed, I'll hear about it tonight." He brushed some lint off his pants and popped gum into his mouth. "Wanna stick?"

"Don't mind if I do."

As they drove through town, Mike painted a mellower bio-sketch of his father. "He's really a great guy. Even before my mother was in the accident, he did everything for us." His voice carried wonderment when he said, "He watches me like a hawk, but I still have room to breathe." He sighed with relief. "He's not like some fathers who live through their kids' accomplishments. He doesn't expect me to be his clone." Laying his head back on the headrest, he told her, "A lot of guys on the team don't even enjoy the game anymore because of all the pressure from Coach Shaffer and some parents."

"I'm sorry to hear that," she said. "Still, it's nice to know you appreciate your father. I know Dr. Wright counts him as a good friend."

Mike nodded. "Most of the time my dad's cool." He let out a laugh and said, "My friends even like being around him because he always teases us. He takes us to car shows and camping." More serious than he needed to be, he added, "Don't get me wrong. He's not a dumb jock or anything. He graduated from Columbia with a business law degree." Sounding content, he said, "We have the most fun at our cabin." Mike cracked his knuckles and let out a nervous laugh. "The only thing wrong with him is he's too particular about women. What're the chances he'll ever find a lady who wants to look at old cars all day, traipse through the wilderness to hunt for supper, and then come home and learn about a thousand-year-old mummy on *The History Channel*?"

Jenna bent her head back and let out a soft laugh. "Don't be too hard on your old man." She gave him a quick side glance before turning her focus back on the road. "Are you familiar with the saying, 'Opposites attract'? Never underestimate the role of chemistry in relationships either. Often people who aren't even looking for a mate will encounter someone who walks into a room, then BAM! They're hooked for life."

She pulled into the banquet hall parking lot and eased up to the entrance. "Have everything you need?"

Mike nodded. "Thanks for helping me out, Miss Rossi."

Winking, she said, "Enjoy the evening, Michael." Before he walked away, she added, "By the way, when your dad lectures you tonight, gently remind him that it's his fault I'm going to look like a Banshee for a week."

Chapter Two

THE PRINCIPAL STROLLED INTO JENNA'S ROOM, PLANTED A memo on her desk, and said, "Looks like Stephen Gaone wants to meet with us." Sitting on the air vent, he asked, "Did you ever meet Steve?"

Jenna typed the last word on a vocabulary quiz, pressed print, and swung around with exaggerated flair to face him. Leaning back in her chair, she said, "No, but I talked with him on the phone."

"You can't find a nicer guy. He has a strong personality, but he's not the least bit self-centered. He's a loyal friend."

She stood and shuffled some papers on her desk. Avoiding eye contact at first, she asked, "Are you going to give me a heads-up? Two students turned in a paper that reads identical to one another. Only your friend wants to usurp my valuable time to dispute the obvious." Looking up, her chin slightly raised, she asked, "Who does Mr. Nice Guy blame for his son's cheating? Me, the rest of the world, or his son?"

Dr. Marcus Wright let out a short laugh. "Paranoia doesn't become you, Jenna. Gaone told me he respects your decision to give both students zeroes. Mike admits he helped Caleb Marawski with the essay, but he swears he had nothing to do with Caleb's actions after he helped him." Narrowing his eyes, he said, "I've never questioned your judgment. Steve Gaone and I are friends, but I won't defend his son's bad behavior; he won't either." Walking toward the door, he turned and said, "You were more than fair with the disciplinary action. All we need to do is be civil and give the Gaones a chance to air their feelings."

She laughed a charming little laugh and said, "Thanks for choosing me over your male pal."

Shrugging, he said, "It's easier to do what's right. Why invite problems?" More philosophical, he said, "People just want to be heard, to be understood. It doesn't cost a lot to listen, but it sure can get expensive in time and legal maneuvering when we don't." As he walked out the door, he said, "Frankly, we have an open and shut case. I'm curious as to what they have to say."

The bell signaled the students to move from the lunchroom to their seventh period classes. Jenna stood outside her classroom near the door and watched Mike Gaone and several of his friends stroll down the hall to her room. Milking the seconds before the tardy bell, the brawny teens congregated in front of the door forcing her to issue a warning.

"Loiter to your heart's content, gentlemen, but understand there's a detention slip with your name on it if you're not in your seat and quiet when that bell rings."

She barely escaped the stampede of sinewy eighteen-year-olds bolting through the narrow doorway all at once. When the tardy bell rang, she mimed an umpire calling a close play, safe!

Candy, a poorly motivated student sporting a head of hair resembling multi-colored grass in a child's Easter basket, asked with her characteristic whine, "Are we doin' anything today, Miss Rossi?"

Before Jenna could address her question, a stocky student in a tight, navy-blue hoodie wrapped both hands around his mouth to form a megaphone. "Earth to Candy, Earth to Candy. Maybe if you'd show up more than once a week, you'd know Rossi's class is the only class we ever work in."

Shooting him a dirty look, Candy turned and stretched her arm across the desk and dropped her head on it.

Jenna seized the opportunity to lecture the students on the benefits of working hard and the cost of taking shortcuts.

"I know you guys find writing assignments challenging, but there are no benefits to selling yourselves short. If you don't learn to research, organize your thoughts to express your ideas, and think for yourselves, expect to have a lot of bosses telling you what to do, and expect to earn less money in your careers." Turning to wipe the board clean, she heard a student mutter a complaint under his breath. She swung around, eyed him, and said, "Life's hard enough, but it's more difficult for poorly educated people."

Alluding to a lesson from the dystopic novel, *Brave New World*, they completed the previous week, Jenna reminded them, "If you opt for a superficial, unintelligent existence, there will always be some intelligent, diabolical person who is more than willing to tell you what to think, what to do, and when to do it." Wiping her hands with a paper towel, she looked up, and asked, "What's so difficult about this class that you believe you can't do the work?"

As though she injected adrenalin into the collective vein of the lethargic class, enthusiastic hands fluttered above their heads like a flock of Canada geese lighting on a pond on an autumn morning.

"The stories are so long," one boy offered.

Holding the bridge of her nose with her thumb and index finger, she closed her eyes for a moment. Her eyes on the tired student again, she watched him yawn wide and long before his body slumped down low into ignorant ease.

Before she could suggest to Eric that it's more mannerly to cover one's mouth when he yawns, an honor student discharging more zeal leaned his chair back, teetered on the hind legs, and said, "You're a good teacher, but those research papers are inhumane." Taking full advantage of his opportunity to vent with little repercussion, he lowered the chair on all fours and continued his confident plea. "Everyone else makes us do one research paper. You make us write three," he said dramatically holding three fingers high over his head. With flair, he pointed and said, "Then you throw those freaky Friday essays at us. They're short, but they take up a chunk of our time." Wagging his finger for emphasis, he summed up saying, "I bet if you check, the Geneva Convention classifies that as torture."

Jenna garnered chuckles when she posed an exaggerated stare at the student and feigned agreement. "Point well made, William. Writing essays is right up there with waterboarding."

Jenna watched as Mike Gaone, who was usually engaging, sat conspicuously silent.

Ahmad, a smart, personable student said, "The truth is your class is harder than most, Miss Rossi, but I really like when we study mythology." He turned to address some of his classmates. "At least she doesn't hate us like Mr. Richland." He swung his eyes back to Jenna. "Richland counts down the days to summer vacation in front of us. You like being around us." He shrugged and said, "We might not like the work, but we like you." Narrowing his eyes, he asked, "Is liking English as much as you do even normal?"

Ahmad's comments drew loud, friendly laughter. Jenna closed one eye, jutted her chin, and said, "Thank you . . . I think . . . for at least noticing that I love being around you guys, Ahmad." With mock indignation, she added, "Just out of curiosity, what does anyone in this class know about normal behavior?" Pointing to the door, she said, "Just ten minutes ago, I watched seven of you mini-sumo wrestlers plow your way through that narrow opening! Call that normal?"

Loud laughter resonated.

The benign tone of the discussion quickly turned malicious when from the back of the room a mean-spirited Caleb Marawski yelled, "Hey Ahmad, the only thing abnormal about Rossi is she actually likes teaching camel-riding, sand flea, Arab terrorists like you."

Caleb's offensive comment earned him the wrath of both teacher and students. Her lifted hand ordered silence from some students who booed his wicked attack. Placing her hands on her hips, she glared at Caleb.

"You sure you're not part rattlesnake? Why so mean?" After a long stare, she softened her tone. "Aren't you part Polish?"

Caleb postured into defensive mode. Piercing her with a cold, penetrating stare, he shot back, "So what?"

"Think, Caleb! Just because Ted Kaczynski's Polish, and he just so happens to be a home-grown convicted terrorist, would you like people to conclude that all Polish people are terrorists?"

Before Caleb could respond, Ken Miller, an arrogant star quarterback, incited an onslaught of laughter by yelling, "Kaczynski's an outlier. Polish people are too dumb to be terrorists."

Caleb sat seething as Jenna swung her eyes to Ken. "Do you see how quickly you guys turned our friendly discussion into an ugly event?" Her glare quieted the room as her narrowed eyes moved from one student to the other.

"Prejudice is never as friendly and fun as we pass it off to be. Belittling a group of people is wrong. Before we know it, every ethnic group is fair game." Her voice carried a plea when she said, "The beauty of America is we're a mixture of nationalities. When we take care of each other, we take care of ourselves." The only sound in the room was an occasional humming of the air vent as she slowly paced from one end of the class to the other, stopping from time to time to make a major point. She engaged each student when she spoke, but her eyes rested on Caleb when she explained, "The best way to protect ourselves from prejudice is to avoid trash-talking and injurious behavior toward people wherever we are, in school, at the movies, and at ball games." As she bent down to pick up a pencil that rolled off a student's desk, she said, "I can't control what happens in the halls or on the street corners, but," she pointed at Caleb and then Ken, "I won't tolerate even a hint of prejudice in this class." She walked toward the far end of the room and cracked open a window. "I'm convinced that if we practice being nice to each other in this room, it will be harder for us to be mean to each other out there." Facing the class, she stressed, "Being nice isn't laughing at someone's racist joke because you don't want to embarrass the person who told the bad joke. Being nice isn't remaining silent because you don't want to offend the perpetrator when his mean words or actions attack another person. Being nice is having the courage to stand up for what's right, even if it means some people might not like you for it." Using capital letters, she printed the word C H A R A C T E R on the board and underlined it twice. Palming the word, she said, "This is what defines genuinely good people!"

Chapter Three

MARCUS WRIGHT SUMMONED JENNA TO HIS OFFICE THE next morning. Bantering on the phone with an irate parent, he waved her in with his free hand.

"For the last time, Mr. Marawski, it doesn't matter that the team needs Caleb to win the game tomorrow night. He should've thought about his team before he delivered that tasteless comment to Mr. Richland. He needs to be more respectful of his teachers and his peers." Marcus rolled his eyes and added, "We both know this isn't exactly Caleb's first ride on the merry-go-round. If he doesn't start exercising good judgment, sitting out a football game will be the least of his problems."

Mr. Marawski hung up.

The principal threw his head back and pointed to the phone. "He thinks we're running a hotel where his kid can check in and out at his convenience. He wants Caleb to serve his suspension after the game." He shoved some papers out of his way. "Talk about team spirit. Coach Shaffer put him up to it!" He covered his face with his hands for a moment, looked up, and tossed his pen on the desk. "In what universe do Shaffer and Marawski believe the world should rearrange rules to accommodate an eighteen-year-old who calls his classmate a sand flea and labels his teacher a fag? All in the name of scoring points for the team!"

"He wins football games," Jenna said. "Caleb is basically a good kid, but when we treat these athletes like royalty, school becomes a breeding ground for entitlement. Little wonder they begin to believe they're above the law." Her tone turned indignant. "Frankly, if I used the same tactics in my classroom as that coach uses on the field—spewing profanity, grabbing them by their necks, and hurling names of female body parts—you'd serve my head up on a silver platter."

Marcus appreciated Jenna Rossi. She was an intelligent, classy, thirty-three-year old woman who surrounded herself with open-minded, fair, and frank friends. She knew how to keep a confidence and fiercely defended people and concepts that she perceived to be grounded in reason. She was petite and attractive. Although personable and vivacious, she artfully disguised a sad component to her that few people detected.

Assured of her friendship, Marcus teased. "You're special. I'd dust off the gold platter for your head."

She stood and curtsied. "Before I leave you, I understand you have a message for me?"

He picked up a note and handed it to her. "It's short notice, but Steve Gaone wants to meet today at four."

She rolled her eyes. "Talk about people wanting life to happen at their convenience." She drew in a deep breath, exhaled, and said, "Let's keep the customer satisfied."

She turned to leave when Marcus said, "I'll call him right now." He shot her an impish grin and asked, "Should I tell him to bring his Porche?"

Narrowing her eyes, she countered, "Only if it means the meeting will end sooner."

The Gaones were first to arrive at the late afternoon meeting. Sitting with his legs crossed, Steve flipped through a magazine that featured vintage automobiles, while his son remained standing, cracking his knuckles, and staring out the window that overlooked the courtyard.

Marcus opened the door to the conference room, extended his hand, and said, "Someday I'll own a Stanley Steamer."

Steve stood, shook hands, and countered, "I'd like to get my hands on a reasonable McLaren F1."

Marcus said, "I'd settle for a ticket to this year's Detroit Auto Show."

Seconds behind Marcus, Jenna entered the room like a gentle wave with just enough force to knock Steve's heart off balance. He struggled not to ogle her.

The plain black dress she wore was sleek and professional. Black, high-heeled sandals accentuated her tanned legs making them look longer than they really were. Curly light brown hair cascaded past her shoulders as her large, hazel-brown eyes welcomed them with sincerity and warmth.

Immediately regretting his failure to reciprocate the earlier favor she afforded his son and him, he felt his heart drifting closer to her and hoped she'd reach out and pull it in.

When Marcus introduced them, she offered Steve a polite wave.

Marcus looked at Steve. "You indicated that Mike wanted to clear the air." He swung his eyes to Mike. "Take as much time as you need, young man."

When Mike glanced at his father, Steve nodded. Mike turned to Jenna and said, "I know it looks like I cheated." He looked at his father and said, "You know I'd never cheat."

Steve nodded his assurance.

Mike swung his eyes back to Jenna. "I just want you to know I only tried to help Caleb. He's worried about college. He asked me to help him write the essay." He shrugged. "So, I explained the poem to him and let him read my paper." He looked down at the notepad in front of him and reasoned, "My father helps me all the time. He reads my papers and gives me ideas. He tells me to choose clearer words or move sentences around." A sheepish smile crossed his lips when he looked up and said, "Sometimes he's worse than you when he crosses out paragraphs and tells me the whole paper's crappy." Staring at Jenna, he asked, "Is that cheating?" His eyes fell on the principal when he said, "My mistake wasn't helping someone. My mistake was when the bell rang, I let Caleb hold onto my paper."

Pausing for several moments, he fixed his gaze on the window across the room overlooking the courtyard. Music and teenage laughter from the cheerleaders practicing their routines at the far end of the hall filtered into the quiet room. More reflective, he said, "Ahmad was right. You're the best teacher we've ever had. I really like your class, and I think you're fair." Clearing his throat, he palmed his chest, and said, "I really care about what you think of me." He turned to the principal. "I wanna be able to ask you guys for recommendations." He swung his eyes back to Jenna. His stare was clear and intense, his voice strong and sincere. "I want you to feel good that you know me. I'm sorry I caused everyone problems." He sat back, looked at his father, and said, "Thanks for hearing me out."

Jenna jotted down a single thought on her notepad, looked up at Marcus, and asked, "May I respond?"

Marcus nodded.

She used the back of her hand to lift her long curly hair off her shoulder. Keeping her voice even and professional, she locked eyes with Mike, and said, "First, I'm impressed with the way you've taken responsibility for your actions, but not surprised." From the corner of her eye, she caught a half-smile cross Steve's lips. Her focus still on Mike, she said, "I'm also convinced your error was bad judgment." She lowered her eyes for several moments and reflected on her own bad judgment in college that derailed part of her life. In a low, more serious voice, she said, "I know adults who are unable to verbalize and reconcile their poor judgment as well as you have in your self-defense." She locked eyes with Mike and said, "The truth is we all exercise bad judgment from time to time, but that doesn't make us bad people."

She swung her eyes to Steve.

The gentle rise and fall of her chest as she breathed evenly and in control captivated him. He couldn't remember the last time he stared into more sincere eyes.

She pulled her hair to one side, smiled, and said, "Dr. Wright tells me you're quite an accomplished person, but after what we just heard this afternoon," she pointed to Mike, "it seems your finest accomplishment is raising this intelligent, articulate, and I'd like to stress, good young man."

Steve suppressed his pounding heart behind a soft, "Thank you."

She lowered her eyes to the yellow legal tablet, tore out the top page, and slid it across the table to Mike. Smiling, she said, "For the record, I really like knowing you." Her eyes grew large, and with more animation she added, "And after this meeting, I even admire your intelligent defense of your good character."

As Marcus stood to adjourn the meeting, Mike silently read the words Jenna scrawled across the page: *GOOD CHARACTER HAS STRENGTH TO ABSORB A FEW BAD JUDGMENTS.*

Steve and Marcus stood at the school entrance conversing like co-conspirators when the soft clicking of heels down the hall forced an abrupt end to their covert discussion. Marcus reached out his hand and said, "Trust your instincts on this one, Steve. She'll add life to your tired, worn out . . . sentences."

A slight wiggle in her hips, she rounded the corner and headed toward Steve. Her self-assured voice teased, "No talkative clients to hold you captive tonight?"

Her attention sent a tingle up his spine as he stood straight, his back up against the brick portion of the wall.

"Mike's at practice; I'm alone tonight."

"No car shows to see? Not even the *History Channel*?" she jabbed with a smile playing on her lips.

Covering his face with his hands, he peeked through his open fingers, and said, "This is what happens when you muzzle the dog instead of your kid." Narrowing his eyes, he asked, "Is there anything my son didn't reveal about me?"

She placed her index finger on her lips and pretended to be in thought. "The last thing he told me was you're destined to remain a bachelor because no woman exists who has that perfect mix of rustic sophistication."

His face reddened. "While I was negotiating with my client, exactly what was my son negotiating with you?"

She bent her head back and let out a laugh. Pointing her index finger at his chest, she said, "The only thing that can drag sensitive information like that out of me is a cheap bottle of wine. Precisely for that reason, I've acquired a fondness for ginger ale."

Reacting with lightning speed to the slight opening she presented, he playfully jumped to one side of her. Slowly, he swept his hand in front of her path and said, "I know a magic place that has all kinds of wonderful wines, and I'll wager it even serves ginger ale for the faint-hearted."

Her eyes widened as heat rushed to her face. Fumbling an apology, she said, "Honest, I wasn't fishing for a dinner date, Mr. Gaone. Mike told me you enjoy teasing people. He also made it clear you don't appreciate women who chase you."

He lifted his chin and looked down at her. "Did Michael detail the exceptions?"

She shook her head.

"Well, Miss Rossi, like the English language, there are exceptions to some Gaone rules." With a glint in his eye, he said, "So, if you're chasing me, it's in my best interest to slow down and be caught."

Playing along, she teased, "You mean until some wealthy client decides to talk you away from me."

He pulled back, raised his arms to his chest, and clenched his fists in front of his face like a boxer poised to protect himself.

"I won't stand idly by while my son and his teacher defame my character." He threw a quick right toward her hand, snatched it, and said, "Come on. I'm going to find a classy place to dine with a classy lady."

They drove for a half hour before he eased onto a cobblestone driveway. At the end of the quarter mile drive, her eyes traveled up the walls of a towering castle named The Renaissance Inn. Lush green grass blanketed the pristine, sprawling hills that surrounded the ancient-looking structure. The soothing, sweet aroma of purple and white butterfly bushes permeated the air. Ivy framed the windows as vines with long green tentacles crawled across the massive gray walls, covering much of the weathered and worn stones. Inside, embers resting in large, rustic, stone fireplaces warmed the vast rooms. Candelabras carrying clusters of candles hovered high above them, casting shadows on the walls. A harp, playing soft and low, accompanied by flutes and violins transported the mind and soul to the days of yore when knights in shining armor rescued damsels in distress.

Her eyes absorbed the magnificence that surrounded her as he ordered a bottle of wine. When the waitress walked away, Jenna asked with awe, "My gosh! How on earth did you find this place?"

The pleasure on her face sent a surge through his body. He admitted, "I didn't."

She swung her eyes to him and said, "You'll never convince me you came by this place accidentally."

Leaning closer to her, he said, "I'll let you in on a secret, but promise you won't tell my son I was talking about him."

She pressed her thumb and index finger together and dragged them across her soft, full lips. "Not a word."

"Mike's been pushing for this meeting ever since you drove him to that banquet." He sat back and gazed at her face. His eyes sparkled when he rendered the opinion, "You can miss every hair appointment for the rest of your life, and you still wouldn't look like a Banshee."

Her mouth dropped. "My gosh! He told you what I said?"

Before he could answer, the waitress promptly placed the wine, two glasses, and a glass of ginger ale on the table, then proceeded to take their order. When she walked away, Steve turned to Jenna and said, "The truth is you're the first woman Mike ever wanted me to dazzle since his mother died, so we had fun one evening researching restaurants with Brit lit names." He gave the room a quick once-over. "We did better than we anticipated."

With slight disappointment, she asked, "So, you invited me here to make Mike happy?"

His arms rested on the table as he massaged his wine glass with both hands. Studying her with thoughtful eyes, he said, "Initially, it seemed an enjoyable way for me to reciprocate the favor you did us." Pointing at her, he added, "The game changed the moment you strolled into that conference room." A soft, "Wow," escaped him. "I knew I had to bring you here." Swirling his wine, he said, "I didn't know it would be tonight." After a brief reflection, he told Jenna, "I had reservations when Mike insisted on that meeting. He was convinced you'd never involve yourself with a man whose son cheated." Setting his glass on the table, he cleared his throat and said, "There's not enough ginger ale in the world to repay you for the way you made my son's heart dance earlier today." He palmed his chest and said, "Hell, you even managed to make *my* heart do the 'Tarantella.'" Patting his breast pocket, he told her, "Mike wanted me to hold onto this 'character' note you gave him. He'll treasure it for the rest of his life."

When she turned her head to stare at the hot flames consuming the log in a fireplace adjacent to their table, he wondered if he had somehow chafed a wound.

Gentle melodies filled the silence between them before she swung her eyes back to him and said, "My parents ingrained the idea of good character in my brother and me ever since we could crawl. My brother never disappointed them. They were devastated when he was killed."

His shoulders slumped. "I'm sorry." After a sip of wine, he asked, "What happened?"

"He was riding home from baseball practice with his friend. His friend's older brother was distracted by the radio. When he ran a stop sign, a pickup truck broadsided them. Five days later, my family gathered to watch my father pull the plug on Josh's life support."

Surprised, Steve said, "I remember my mother talking about that accident." His face visibly pained, he searched her face and asked, "That was your brother?"

"That was Josh."

"Did they charge the driver?"

Her eyes watered for only a second. Clearing her throat, she said, "My father advocated leniency. He didn't want to burden Josh's memory with a ruined life."

Steve raised his brows. "I thought only God forgives that mightily."

"I resented my dad until the day I learned that Mark Packard makes the world a better place."

Steve's eyes narrowed. "Doctor Mark Packard, the psychiatrist who works wonders with vets suffering from post-traumatic stress disorders?"

Jenna nodded.

Gently scratching a speck of dried food off the table with her finger, she said, "Not a day goes by that I don't think of Josh. He never caused my parents a moment of worry." Raising her eyes, she added with more levity, "I, on the other hand—"

Interrupted by her phone, she glanced at the caller's name. "Excuse me. I always take Sam's calls."

Widening his eyes, he masked his resentment of the interloper, and asked, "Do you need privacy with him?"

Holding Steve's eyes with a steady gaze, she said, "Sam, you know I love you, but it's an inconvenient time. I'm with the father of a student."

Steve's jaw tightened.

A disgruntled Sam complained, "At least you picked up. I wanna call my analyst, but the idiot . . . The asshole never answers my calls. I'm not goin' back. She was so wonderful when I first met her. I know why, too. She wanted somethin'. All she does is take and take and take my money. What do I get? Fuckin' flashbacks that make me want to kill someone."

"You need a doctor that specializes in abuse cases, Sam."

"Great! I'ma case now." She let out a loud burp and added, "Keep tellin' me what I need, Jen. 'You need this, Sam. You need that, Sam. Go ta church. Volunteer. Stand up. Sit down. Fight, fight, fight.' Well I'm tired of fighting!" Screaming, she said, "When you gonna come help me do all the things you think I need to do, Jen?"

"Calm down, Samantha."

Steve tilted his head as a half-smile began to play on his lips.

Louder, Sam said, "No one picks up. Robots, mechanical voices all day long. They're so busy with their selfish lives. Can't even answer a damn phone." Pouting, she mumbled, "Whocares anyway?"

"I care, but I can't talk right now."

Sam's tone turned belligerent. "Yeah, right!" After a short pause, she asked with a loud voice carrying over to Steve, "Is he screwing you? That's what he really wants, Jen. For God's sake," she wailed, "Puhleeze . . . Don't let him screw you! Don't let him . . ." Her voice drowned in sobs.

Jenna's face reddened as she insisted, "That won't be happening tonight. I gotta go."

"Wait, wait, wait," Sam pleaded. "Don't get mad." She hiccupped before stuttering, "I did . . . didn't mean it."

With unnatural calm, Jenna said, "I'm not mad, but I'm being rude talking on the phone while he's sitting across from me."

"We wouldn't want ta be rude to our friends, would we?" Sam asked full of resentment before hanging up abruptly.

Exhaling an exaggerated breath, Steve eyed Jenna, and asked, "What was that all about?"

"We grew up together. Her parents used her as a punching bag, and I'm the only one who still listens."

He sipped some wine, shook his head, and feigned disappointment. "So, tonight we're not . . ."

Embarrassed by her failed attempt to camouflage Sam's inordinate fear, there was a hint of sorrow behind her soft smile when she said, "It'll take more than a fairy-tale dinner in a magnificent castle with a dashing gentleman for me to . . ." She looked away for a second before swinging her eyes back to him. "You have excellent taste in restaurants."

"Aha," he said, with a twinkle in his eyes. "Maybe I'll have better luck with this question. What kind of troublemaking kid did your parents have to—"

Her raised hand stopped him. With more levity, she said, "Let's save the details of my oppositional defiant youth for the second date, okay?"

He rubbed his open hands together with enthusiasm. "That was easy!"

With a deadpanned look, she asked, "You think I'm easy?"

"Not at all," he said, maintaining his excitement. "It took time to orchestrate a first date, and tonight unfolded easier than expected. Now you're proposing a second date before this one's even over."

"You said it again," she teased.

Tilting his head, he said, "You're about as easy as deciphering the first three words of *Genesis*, Rossi." He let out a short laugh. "Just when I think I know what 'In the beginning' means, some highfalutin theologian comes along and asks, 'In the beginning of what?'"

Losing the battle to feign insult, her lips curved into a smile. "Mike was right."

He drank some wine and asked, "About what?"

"You're far from being a dumb jock."

"Studying at Columbia will do that to a person." He sipped more wine and said, "That university wasn't easy or cheap. God knows being married and raising a kid didn't make it any easier."

"I bet you graduated in the top ten of your class."

"A little better than that."

"Really?"

"Your amazement insults me, Rossi."

Defending herself, she said, "You have to admit, top ten in a kindergarten class would be impressive. Top five at Columbia given your circumstances? Give me a break!" Sweeping his face, she stopped to study the lines around his eyes that conjured character. "I socialize with some brilliant people. Not one of them would need prompting to boast if he owned the academic bragging rights that you do." Her eyes grew large. "If I graduated in the top five of my class, the Rossi clan would've pawned everything they owned, including my grandfather's prosthetic leg, to rent every billboard in town." Eyeing him, she asked, "So?"

"So, what?" he countered.

"So, what number were you, hot shot?"

Before he had a chance to answer, she waved her hand and said in mock disgust, "I'm probably conversing with a Columbia University valedictorian, right?"

"Since academic standing seems important to you, Jenna, let's make this fair and fun." Soft and seductive, he said, "Show me yours; I'll show you mine."

Palming her face with one hand, she said, "You're trying to embarrass me."

"You mean the way you've been embarrassing me for the past five minutes?" He motioned for her to 'come on' and reveal her class standing. When she balked, he suggested, "Would it be less painful if we write it down?"

She hesitated at first, then reached for a paper napkin. Sitting up straight, pretending to gather the courage she needed to perform the Herculean task before her, she said, "Okay, let's do this. Get ready; get set; go!"

With slight hesitation, she slipped her napkin bearing number eleven across the table.

"Not too shabby, Miss Rossi."

She stared at his neatly printed number four for several seconds before looking up.

"Obviously, I spoke in haste when I said this ginger ale makes us even. I was unaware that you had more to offer than money, status, and charm."

Captivated by her playful spirit, he placed his elbows on the table, clasped his hands, and said, "I'm in the presence of a rarity, a woman who appreciates qualities in a guy besides the cash he carries."

Pulling back, she said, "We exist." With more levity, she added, "Considering I saved the lives of two Gaone men in one evening and that brain of yours is bursting with brilliance, I think it's only fair you teach me at least half of what's in that smart-alecky head of yours."

"That may take more than a second date," he countered with a wry grin. Pouring some Chardonnay into her empty wine glass, he said, "Let's begin tonight with lesson number one: how humans come to be."

She gently pushed the wine aside, reached for her ginger ale, and said, "How intriguing. I thrive on theological discussions."

"I was thinking biology."

"No, Mr. Columbia. How people come to be is theology. God calls people into being." Her smile teased when she added, "You did admit *Genesis* baffles you."

Challenging her claim, he asked, "If what you say is true, why do colleges require OB/GYNs to study biology rather than theology?"

Initially stumped by his assertion, she asked, "Are you trying to catch me in an intellectual trap?"

Eyeing her seductively, he told her, "If I do manage to catch you," he sipped some wine, "in an intellectual trap or otherwise, I'd be a happy man."

To mask her excitement at the prospect of being caught by the handsome specimen sitting across from her, she massaged the glass in her hands and acquired a professorial tone.

"Let's get back to the discussion. God calls humans into being. OB/GYNs simply act as knowledgeable agents of delivery." Winking, she said, "I know my theology and biology, Mr. Gaone." She added, "Don't let that number eleven on my transcript lull you into underestimating my cognitive ability."

Subtly rebuking her bravado, he countered, "I know I don't know everything, so maybe you need to share that brain burgeoning with knowledge with me."

She let out a spontaneous laugh. "I'm not as arrogant as I sound. I'm just doing a lousy job acting like I'm as smart as you really are." She dipped a piece of bread into the olive oil mixture and said with confidence, "I'll teach you all I know about literature, and you teach me more about theology and biology." Shooting him a disarming smile, she asked, "Will that work?"

His eyes, wide and excited, he said, "Throw in a Sunday dinner date with kalamata olives, and it's a deal."

Pulling back in surprise, she said, "Oh my gosh! You like kalamata olives?"

His heart danced at the sound of her voice rhythmically describing her favorite olive dish.

"I cut up fresh tomatoes, roasted red peppers, and olives." She seductively ran her tongue over her lips and said, "It's to die for." She held up her hand, palm facing him and said, "Crushed, juicy garlic sautés in olive oil making the whole house smell like an Italian bistro. All the ingredients blend with the seasonings in that savory oil." Pointing at him, she said with excitement, "I boil angel hair pasta and top it with pieces of plump, juicy, grilled chicken breasts sprinkled with feta."

"Feta?" he asked.

She bunched together her fingers on one hand, brought them to her lips, and smacked them with a soft kiss. "You can't get enough of it!"

I can't get enough of you, he thought, but he told her, "You own Sunday afternoon."

Wiping her fingers with a napkin, she asked, "Are you always so accommodating?"

He reminded her, "Mike didn't believe I was so accommodating the day you drove him to the banquet." With dismay, he said, "I don't like saying 'no,' but what does a guy do when he's pulled in several directions at the same time?"

"The word *no* is problematic for students, too," Jenna said.

More seriously than she anticipated, Steve told her, "The concept of no is more complicated than the two simple letters suggest. Look at the *Just Say No* campaigns. They're superficial and even damaging in some cases." Pausing for several seconds, he asked, "How do we expect teenagers to just say no to vices on a Friday night when they see adults around them indulging in the same bad practices? The kids know they'll be ostracized by their peers in the cafeteria on Monday." Wiping his mouth with a napkin, he said, "The emotional and psychological toll of ostracism isn't any easier for adults either. Just last month I had a business meeting where a lucrative contract hinged on whether I engaged in a threesome with the client and his nymphomaniac wife."

Jenna's eyes widened. "Oh my gosh. You lost the contract because you said 'no' to perverted sex?"

"No way was I going to lose that contract!"

Her shoulders slumped. She sat back and stared at him with mild detachment. Before she irrevocably cooled, Steve said, "I told the guy I was a born-again virgin, that I was saving myself for marriage. Fortunately, he found me funny and didn't push it. He signed on with me despite my refusal to play with him and his promiscuous, albeit attractive, wife."

She broke into a warm, relieved smile. "The way you were talking, it sounded like—"

"Like I'm just another rich guy willing to sell his soul for money?"

"I'm sorry if I made you feel like I was judging you."

Pointing at her, he said, "You did judge me, and I learned something important about you."

Not sure she wanted to hear how she gave him reason to second guess her enthusiasm for him, she welcomed the waitress serving their food and engaged her with small talk.

"I really like that waitress. She does her job well."

"Why, Miss Rossi, aren't you the slightest bit curious about what it is I learned about you?"

"Maybe a little."

"I learned your soul's not for sale either."

Tapping his index finger on the table, he said, "There's no mistaking your body language. Had I engaged in that threesome, this night was going to end early, and you'd be battling a chronic case of 'fakasia.'"

Puzzled, she asked, "What's 'fakasia'?"

"A fake illness that attacks you every time I call."

Letting out a short laugh, she said, "I'm going to come down with 'fakasia' the next time I have a parent / teacher conference."

"There's a better disease for skipping work. Claim a case of 'anal glaucoma.'"

"Gosh, that sounds fatal."

"It's not a physical disease; it's more attitudinal. People habitually can't see reasons to drag their butts to work."

Laughing, she told him, "You're quite entertaining. I'm glad you didn't equate my initial wavering to have dinner with you tonight with a *no*."

"You showed enough interest to inspire me."

"So, if you wanted something badly enough and someone said 'no,' would you walk away or would you fight for it?"

Folding his napkin and pushing it to the side, he said, "It depends. It's easier to force my hand in business." He perused her face and said, "My family showered me with love my whole life. It seems unnatural to fight for it." He broke into a broad smile.

"What's so funny?"

With both elbows on the table, he clasped his hands and told her, "When I was ten years old, my dad drove me to the pound to adopt a dog. He taught me an important lesson about relationships that day." Nursing his wine, he said, "My dad told me it didn't matter if I liked every dog in the joint. The only pup worth taking home was the one that followed me around." He poured more wine into his glass and offered her some.

"No, I'm good."

"So, we're walking around the pound, and I asked my dad what would happen if the dog that followed me wasn't the best dog in the pound? He looked me dead in the eye and said, 'Stevie, if it's following you, then that dog wants to be with you. If you surround yourself with animals and people who want to be with you, you'll never have to wonder where their loyalties lie. That makes them the best for you.'" Steve lifted his glass as though he were making a toast.

Holding his gaze, she said, "I'm wondering why a confident man wants to hook up with a woman who follows him around like a puppy."

Playing with her eyes, he said, "The ideal would be a shapely creature, with curly brown hair, and confidence to challenge me for my own good." He leaned back in his chair. "Difficult to attain," with a softer voice, "even more difficult to let go."

"Why would you let go?" Jenna asked, blushing, but still playing along.

"I wouldn't want to let go, but if she wants to follow someone else. . ." His eyes fell to the table. "If she wants to be with someone else . . ." He looked up and locked eyes with her. "I'd have to let go."

Rescuing him from elaboration, the waitress approached the table to ask about their satisfaction with the dinners.

As Steve complimented the waitress on the atmosphere of the inn and on her cheerful demeanor, Jenna rested her chin in the palm of her hand and vacantly stared into the formless flames dancing in the fireplace. Steve's voice sounded distant as he asked several questions about the ownership and the amount of business the inn experienced on a weekly basis.

Swept up in the fantasy of him, Jenna felt his taut arms gather her in. He drew her so close that her firm breasts flattened against his hard chest. His breath was hot on her neck as her heart pounded in rhythm with his. His lips wended their way across her face, gently nibbling at her cheeks, then her chin, until they locked with slight force on her quivering lips. He pressed down hard and lingered long. His relentless tongue wedged its way between her closed lips and swept her into wild ecstasy. Unable to subdue the sensation rising in her, the masculine smell of him thrust her on the verge of losing control. Gasping for air, she—

"Jenna!"

His voice jolted her out of thought. Flustered, she fumbled to conceal the explicit imaginings that she gradually realized he couldn't possibly see. Forcing a nervous smile, she said, "It's so easy to get lost in the majesty of this place." Glancing away for several seconds, she caught his knowing gaze from the corner of her eye. More composed, she held a bite of her meal close to her lips and asked, "Are all your dates this unique?"

Playing with a spoon, he said, "Not really." Raising his chin, he said, "I have to admit, you're the first to go MIA right before my eyes." He studied her for a moment before asking with playful accusation, "Wherever you were, was it nice?"

Dabbing her lips with a napkin, she said, "You have a talent for turning the innocent into lewdness."

Playfully bobbing his head back and forth, he countered, "Guilty as charged," adding "Did you ever wonder what the world would be like if people had thought-bubbles hovering over their heads?"

Rolling her eyes, she said, "We'd all end up being embarrassed to death and hating each other."

"What would my reaction be to the bubble over your head a few seconds ago?"

More serious than she intended, she told him, "I hope I never give you reason to hate me."

Settling back, he said, "To your original question; my dates are few and uneventful." His eyes brightened with mischief when he added,

"Unless I count the time I had dinner with this gorgeous blonde who wouldn't stop ripping on RuPaul."

"RuPaul, the drag queen?"

"The one and only." Raising his hand to the bridge of his nose, he said, "I had it up to here with her gender trash talk for over three quarters of the evening."

Her eyes large with interest, she asked, "How'd you manage to change the subject?"

"I suggested RuPaul looks better than most of my dates." With an air of innocence, he claimed, "Who knew she'd over-react like a psychotic mixing her meds."

"What did you expect after that insinuation?"

An impish grin danced on his mouth. He sipped his wine and pleaded outlaw-wise. "Would a secure woman take that comment personally?" Comically imitating her reaction, he said, "She flung her napkin on the table, yanked her Louis Vuitton handbag resembling a carry-on suitcase, and screeched, 'I don't care how much money Sadie says you have. You're an ignorant, arrogant bastard!'" He waved his hand back and forth over the table. "It took about thirty seconds for the smoke billowing over my head to clear. As the smell of smoldering pride lingered, every eye in that restaurant was staring at me."

After a robust laugh, Jenna cleared her throat and asked in her teacher voice, "Now, Stephen, what did you learn from that experience?"

Narrowing his eyes, he said, "Compare your date to RuPaul. If she walks out, consider yourself lucky because she's insecure. Chances are, she won't tolerate too much else you do."

"Isn't that a bit cynical?"

"Not at all. I married a woman I barely knew because I had to. I was just a kid, and I thought my life was over," he snapped his fingers, "like that!" He poked a piece of cucumber with his fork, popped it into his mouth, and chewed for several moments. Brushing his napkin across his lips, he said, "Don't get me wrong; we both loved Mike. We simply weren't Hallmark material." Finishing up his meal, he told her, "My parents wanted me to stay single and just pay child support, but Amy made all kinds of threats if I didn't marry her. I never really knew her, so romantic love was never a factor between us. We cultivated a friendship and muddled through some rough times, but I was keenly aware she stayed with me because I took care of her. Mike gave us good reason to stick it out."

Jenna caught a hint of sadness in his eyes before he looked down and stared at his wine glass. A soft sigh escaped him before he raised his eyes and said, "After Amy died, I vowed I'd never . . . I won't ever live like that again." Leaning back in his chair, he asserted, "It would be nice if the next Mrs. Gaone tingled when I touched her." With a warm smile, he added, "I'd like to tingle, too."

The waitress interrupted the awkward silence by clearing the empty plates from their table and placing the bill near Steve.

Unsure of how to react to his honest appraisal of his marriage, Jenna said, "I didn't mean to stir unpleasant memories."

"You were teasing, and I threw a curve ball." He pointed to her ginger ale. "Maybe if I were drinking that stuff, I wouldn't talk so much."

Raising her glass, she said, "I learned the hard way that soft drinks go better with good judgment."

He leaned closer, propped his elbows on the table, and clasped his hands. "We're back to that Rossi mystery."

Tracing the rim of her glass with her finger, she said, "I shudder to think how many Rossi secrets I'd divulge if this were any stronger."

His gaze was intense, his voice serious. "This wine isn't the reason I confided in you, Jenna, and that ginger ale isn't the reason why you won't confide in me."

Her smile siphoned the chill out of the cool night air as he walked her to her car in the school parking lot. Before she turned to slip into the driver's seat, he grabbed her arm and told her, "I don't want to wait until Sunday to see you again."

Pretending to straighten his tie, she said, "I know what you really want."

His voice soft and low, he said, "You know better than that."

She laughed saying, "Admit it! You want another chance so you can compare me to some transvestite who's probably prettier than I am."

Grazing her cheek with the back of his hand, he said, "You, Miss Rossi, are in a class by yourself."

Batting her eyelashes, she fanned herself, and imitated a southern belle saying, "Why, Mr. Gaone! I do feel faint. I don't know if I can withstand a brilliant Columbia University graduate complimenting me with the most worn teacher cliché of the century."

"Before the frail lady faints, she should acknowledge truth never ages and needs no adornment; false flattery and faddish comparisons do."

They laughed together as he held her hand and played with her fingers. "It's not as impressive as The Renaissance Inn, but I'd love to take you to Mike's game tomorrow night. We can share a drink with some friends afterward."

Within seconds, her closeness cooled. She told him, "I'm not ready to be on display in front of students and their parents."

"People generally hide when they're ashamed of what they're doing." Searching her face, he asked, "Are you ashamed to be seen with me?"

"Don't be silly. Try to see it from my point of view. Being a teacher is different than being a businessman. Business people sit in restaurants any time, day or night, and people assume they're talking business. If I were in a bar at one in the morning talking to my insurance man, the next day I'd be a twitter sensation. It doesn't take much to ruin a reputation."

Confusion crossed his face. "I'm not asking you to sit with me in a bar at one o'clock in the morning. I'm asking you to sit with me on high school bleachers under bright lights to cheer on kids you teach every day in class."

She countered, "Dating the father of one of my students can spawn some awkward moments."

"For the sake of clarity, are you telling me our relationship has to be covert? I don't slink in the shadows well."

Rolling her eyes, she said, "Stop making it sound so clandestine. I'm only asking for a few weeks of discretion. If we find ourselves incompatible, we can part without all the brouhaha."

His head told him to let it go for another day, but his heart wanted to be with her, and she was saying 'no' to him. Against reason, he escalated the stand-off.

He crossed his arms over his chest and asked, "Does popularity matter that much to you?"

Fighting the hot mist blurring her vision, she said, "I guess they didn't teach connotation at Columbia. There's a chasm between popularity and respect." Struggling to maintain composure, she added, "I'm sorry you view desire for respect as a character flaw, but it's difficult for me to be indifferent to how my students and their parents view me, how I view myself." She brushed her wet cheek with her open hand. "I have another flaw, too. I'm rambling like your self-indulgent clients who keep you longer than you care to be with them."

Before he could assure her that all he wanted was to be with her until night turned into day, she slipped into her car and drove away.

Standing in the empty parking lot, he spun around and slammed the palm of his hands on the top of the car. He bent his head back, peered into the night sky, and whispered with recrimination, "How'd I let magic dissolve into tears?" The wind picked up, carrying a chill that seeped to his bones. Besides his aching heart longing to make the evening right again, the only other sounds were the flurry of chirping tree frogs and an occasional car speeding up the desolate road.

Mike bounded down the stairs and jumped the last two steps.

"What happened, Dad? How'd she like the restaurant?"

Disguising the dismal climax of the evening, he told him, "She was impressed."

Pumping his father for more information, his face brightened when he asked, "Impressed enough to see you again?"

He didn't have the heart to tell his eager son he made her cry. Instead, like a politician managing a crisis that threatened his favorability rating, he put the best positive spin on the debacle and hoped to buy time to stop the slide.

"We need to work a few bugs out." He chugged some water, wiped his mouth with his fingers, and said, "Don't say anything to her about tonight. I'd like to keep school life and private life separate."

Reading between the lines, Mike had no interest in forcing his father to admit failure. Harnessing his enthusiasm, he said, "No problem, Dad. I hope things work out."

"Thanks, Mike. See you in the morning."

Steve climbed the stairs slower than usual. He lingered in the shower, but no amount of hot water cascading over his body could wash away the image of Jenna's glistening eyes. All he could do for now was roll into bed and pray he'd get a chance to make it right.

Chapter Four

MIKE TAPPED JENNA ON THE SHOULDER AND SAID, "ME and Ty loaded up the boxes. If you don't need us for anything else, we're takin' off."

With a smile, Jenna emphasized, "*Ty and I,*" then quickly added, "This library fundraiser would've been in trouble without all you guys." After a swift survey of the room, she came back to them, winked, and said, "Scram before I find more work for you to do."

Mike called his father to let him know that he was hitching a ride with friends.

Steve said, "I'm just around the corner. I'll catch you at home."

Mike cupped his mouth and whispered, "If you're that close, Dad, pick us up. Rossi's still here tallying the proceeds from the sale."

"Stalking her's not a promising idea."

"Come on, Dad. Just say 'hi' and see what happens."

Waving the paper money high above her head, Jenna announced, "One thousand, five hundred, thirty dollars, and twenty-five cents!"

A loud cheer rose from the small group mingling and picking on leftover snacks from the refreshment table.

When Steve slipped through the door, his eyes rolled around the room before settling on Jenna sitting high on a stool with her legs crossed, her back to the door. In deep concentration, she placed the money and the paperwork, completed in triplicate, in a leather bag. He hovered close behind her.

Careful not to attract attention, he grazed his lips close to her ear and whispered a quick, "Hi."

She swung around. Her legs still crossed caused her foot, sporting bright red nail polish, to brush against the calf of his leg. It sent a tingling sensation through his body. Visibly surprised at the sight of him, she greeted him with a friendly, "Well hello!"

"I'm having trouble curbing my enthusiasm," he whispered. "I don't want people to get the impression I'm thrilled to see you."

More reserved, she countered, "I don't expect you to understand."

Before she could swing around and use her paperwork to ignore him, he said, "You have every right to expect a person who says he cares about you to understand how you feel."

Sitting taller, she asked, "Are you going to the away game this Friday? I hate to miss it, but that traffic is awful."

He perused her from head to toe and made her fidget.

After the remaining parent volunteers cleaned up and waved goodbye, he swung his eyes to where his son waited for him outside the door. Casually pulling his keys from his pocket, he turned with a playful leer, and said, "Ride with me at your own risk."

She let out a short laugh. "I've encountered some unsavory people, Stephen." Tilting her head, she added, "You're not one of them."

Eyeing her he countered, "I'll guarantee your safety on the way to the game, but I plan to take full advantage of these," he tapped her lips, "on the way home."

His precocious gesture robbed her of speech for only a moment. She slid off the stool and boasted, "These lips may look girly, cowboy, but they can take anything these," she touched his lips, "can dish out." Placing her hands on her hips, she bragged, "I'm so tough, I can outride most men on a mechanical bull." Polishing her nails on her shoulder, she added, "I clocked eight and a half seconds last summer at the Spartan County Fair!"

His jaw dropped. Unable to resist the tease, he countered, "Anyone can ride a mechanical bull, Miss Rossi. The true test is one's performance on a live bull."

Her mouth gaped. Blood rushed to her face like mercury in a thermometer registering heat at high noon. Pronouncing her words with deliberation, she said, "I can't. . . believe. . . I waltzed into that one." She rolled her eyes and playfully commanded, "Get out before you strip me of all dignity."

"Do we really want to discuss stripping in front of them?" he motioned his head toward the two boys milling outside the door.

Before she could counter, he opened the door to leave.

"Mr. Gaone! The ginger ale's on me."

Flashing a broad smile, he motioned a thumbs-up and walked away.

"What was that all about, Dad?"

"Your teacher wants to hitch a ride to the game."

"Yeah, right," Ty chimed in. "There's a target on your back, Mr. G, and she's aiming for it."

"What makes you so sure she doesn't simply need a ride?"

"Rossi's never missed one of our games. A cool dude like you shows up, and now she needs a ride?" Ty laughed. "She's after you, but at least she's hot."

Mike threw Ty a cautionary look.

Quick to discern Mike's cue, Ty added, "Don't get me wrong, Mr. Gaone. She's a great lady. Talk to her about *Beowulf* and Chaucer. You'll have her wrapped around your finger. Just don't tell any dirty jokes or make fun of anyone's last name. No matter how cool you are, she'll walk and won't look back."

"How is it that you're an expert on Miss Rossi's likes and dislikes?"

"Geez, Mike. Talk to your old man." He told Steve, "She lectures us every time someone makes fun of anyone. We can't say the word *retard* or call someone a fag without her goin' off on us. Talk about someone's slanted eyes, and she'll straighten your thinking out real fast."

Mike laughed and asked, "Remember when Ahmad forgot to write that imagery paper?" Palming his chest, he laughed harder. "He tried to make Rossi forget to collect the essays by saying Aung San Suu Kyi's eyes looked funny."

They bantered and laughed for over a minute before Ty said, "Rossi lectured us about diversity for over half the period then collected the papers right before the bell rang!"

Mike proclaimed, "Nothing beats that day she nailed Marawski for calling Ahmad a sand flea terrorist."

"Retards, fags, and sand fleas, huh? All you need is a set of white sheets, a cross, and a box of matches. Out of all the words in the English language, why choose words designed to hurt? Negative connotations don't help forward a discussion. Practice using language that gets your point across without degrading and polarizing people."

Mike rolled his eyes.

Ty said, "She could've been our math teacher, then we'd really have problems."

Mike burst out laughing.

"Hey, guys, character counts. Maybe there's more depth to your teacher than meets your juvenile eyes."

"Man, how'd we suddenly become juveniles, Dad? We're just tellin' you what she's like. We didn't say anything mean. We like the lady."

"If you guys would stop dragging your knuckles long enough, maybe you'd pick up the point she's trying to make."

"Now we're cave men? Tell us more about using nicer words, Dad."

"It's a good thing we're almost home," Ty said, unbuckling his seatbelt and sliding onto the car floor. He cried out, "Help! Get me out of the Gaone car. I'm regressing into a juvenile. No, no, I mean a Neanderthal."

Steve parked the car in the driveway, turned to the boys, and said with a smirk, "You two are poster boys for accelerating space exploration. There needs to be some place out there where we could train thirteen to nineteen-year-olds to be civil before we invite them back to live on Earth."

"No offense Dad, but maybe that planet would work better for the over thirties. We juveniles didn't crucify Christ, cause slavery, and we don't cause all the wars."

Steve stood speechless as Mike and Ty high-fived each other and walked into the house.

Chapter Five

UNSEASONABLY CHILLY WEATHER DIDN'T STOP SPARTAN supporters from packing the stadium to capacity. Huddling close to keep warm, die-hard fans jumped to their feet energizing themselves each time the team threatened to score. Steve coaxed Jenna to keep herself wrapped in his red and black, wool blanket, insisting that he could handle the chill. When he did sit beside her, he exercised care with the public displays of affection. He had no desire to rekindle the flames of discontent he managed to douse.

Several minutes remained on the clock as droves of fans hoping to beat the traffic poured from the bleachers. The result was a traffic jam in the parking lot.

Disappointed, Jenna said, "It'll be late by the time we get back to Sparta. Will Mike be okay?"

"My mother and father volunteered to catch him at that end."

A car horn blared as one driver spewed profanity at another driver who cut ahead of the others waiting their turn to exit the lot. Steve mumbled, "And people want to know why we can't negotiate world peace." His jaw tightened as he ran his hand through his hair. "These jackasses can't even empty a high school parking lot with civility." Turning to Jenna, he apologized. "This certainly wasn't part of my plan."

"I thought there was only one item on your agenda," she said, with a tease.

He leaned back in the driver's seat, reached for her hand, and played with her fingers. Peering into the night sky, he said, "I wanted to get back early enough to drive to one of the highest points in the city, look up at the stars, and . . ." His unfinished thought hung in the air like bait on a hook.

"And?"

Sharing amusement at the thought, he told her, "The kids offered me romance advice. Tyler suggested that if I talk *Beowulf* and Chaucer, you'd follow me around forever."

"Really?" she asked, fumbling her phone.

"Who you calling?"

"I'm calling the guru of love to advise him that if he'd talk *Beowulf* and Chaucer to me, he'd graduate with the rest of his class."

He pretended to wrestle the phone from her and said, "Leave the poor kid alone. He just wants to see me happy."

Jabbing him with her elbow, she said, "He's not the only one interested in making you happy."

"Hmmm," he said softly. Playing with her fingers again, he asked, "How does the classy lady plan to make me happy?"

Ignoring his lure, she glanced at her watch and complained. "Since when is emptying a parking lot such an ordeal?" Looking up, she asked, "No matter how late it is when we get back, will you take me to the highest point?"

He warned, "Magic happens up there."

With a hint of sadness, she said, "Magic never lasts."

"Then you've never experienced real magic."

He parked the car high on the hill and leaned back on the hood. She backed up into him and rested warm and secure in his arms. The cold, night air was still as they gazed out over the city flickering with bright lights.

"How could I live here all my life and not know this place existed?" she asked, mesmerized by the panoramic view.

Resting his chin on top of her head, he said, "I discovered this spot last year when a client planned to build a house on this property. The deal fell through, so I bought the land for myself."

She twisted around and asked, "You own this hill?"

Nodding, he said, "The real prize is my cabin, but this is a close second." Holding her tighter, he said, "Only the male species in my family visits the cabin, but I'll make an exception for you on our seventh date."

"What's so special about a seventh date?"

Brushing his cheek on her earlobe, he said, "I need time to convince the thirty-pound snapping turtle not to take a chunk outta your beautiful, bare leg when we go skinny dipping in the lake."

She stared at him wide-eyed. Shaking her head, she said, "I don't care how much money Sadie says you have; there's no way you'll get me to dive into a scum-filled pond that's home to snapping turtles. And from what little you know of me, do I remotely fit the profile of the skinny-dipping type?" She gave him an animated stare for several seconds, then turned to gaze at the city below.

Burying his face between her neck and ear, he whispered, "We'll settle all that later. Right now, I get to hold you as close and as long as I want." He turned her around to face him and made an exaggerated sweep of the area. "No eyes or tongues around to feed the rumor mill, and if I want to see fireworks, I can even do this." He gently cupped her face and planted a soft kiss on her lips that gradually turned more passionate. Lingering for several moments, he brushed his mouth to her ear and whispered, "Nothing like the Fourth of July, but—"

Her heart sank. Wounded by his flippant comment, she pulled back and asked, "What's wrong with you? I waited all evening. I waited weeks for this moment." Freeing herself from his arms, she asked, "Is everything a joke to you?"

He pulled back. Looking over one shoulder and then the other, he asked, "Are you sure you're talking to the right guy?" Palming his chest, he said, "I know I can be a wise-guy at times, but I'm the one who scoured the countryside for a fairy tale restaurant to impress you. I'm the same guy who drove you to the top of this hill that overlooks the whole city so that you'd always remember our first kiss." He pointed at her and said, "A place, I might add, so special to me that I've never considered sharing it with any woman but you." He stepped away from her to blow off steam. Shuffling back, he asked, "And you have the audacity to question my serious regard for romance?" He turned away and yelled out over the city, "I can't win with this lady!"

A deep, agonizing groan escaped him as he watched her turn away and cross her arms over her chest, partly to keep warm, partly to shield herself from his mounting frustration. He wanted to understand her ambivalence toward him, but she closed up as tight as a water lily at dusk.

He looked at her with pleading eyes. "Before I take you home, do I get a chance to complete my flippant thought?"

Biting her bottom lip to keep it from shaking, she glanced at him sideways and asked, "Why is a little sensitivity too much to ask from any of you hungry hounds?"

"So, that's what this is about? You're comparing me to the worst in your love life?"

He reached out saying, "Come here." Pulling her closer, he felt a slight shiver move through her body. He whispered, "It's not the Fourth of July, but I swear every one of those bright stars danced across the sky when my lips touched yours, a dazzling prelude for what we have in store for each other." Turning her toward the city below, he pointed, and said, "See all those houses down there; most of them are filled with people who share beds. They raise children; they amass fortunes, but they're sailing through thick fog without a harbor in sight." After a pause, he continued, "They're searching for someone or something to fill them, but they'll never find it." He pressed his cheek to hers. "They're afraid of being rejected." Holding her closer, he said, "I lived that fear." He kissed her ear and whispered, "I finally found a heart that doesn't flash like a cold, neon sign lighting up a fast-food restaurant. I feel alive when I'm with you. You're the passion missing in my life, and I don't want to lose it. I don't want to lose you."

His plea melted the frosty barrier she had forged since her college days. She turned to face him and said, "You did everything right, and I did it wrong." Her voice cracked. "It's like my whole life's built on a block of sand. I'm always watching everything I want, everything I love get washed away." Looking off to the side, she wiped her wet face with her hands. "The last time I tingled when a guy touched me, I had to give up so much of myself." Her lower lip quivered as she crossed her arms, turned, and gazed out over the city.

"I'm a different guy, Jenna, and I sure as hell didn't do everything right. Whatever mistakes we've made, we're older and wiser people. We're standing high on this hill tonight because our hearts want to soar."

Kicking a small mound of dirt in front of her, she faced him and said, "I trusted a guy once, and not even three minutes after he . . ." She looked away. "He zipped up his jeans, grabbed me, and practically shoved me out of his apartment." She glanced at him sideways and asked, "What do you think the Spartan seniors and their parents would think if they knew that tidbit about their airbrushed teacher?"

Holding her, he said, "All I know is a beautiful woman convinced my son that character is a series of good acts, not an isolated mistake. That lady's a keeper in my book."

A rare contentment filled her as she let herself believe his heart and mind were sympathetic to her flaws. She stood on the tips of her toes and planted a soft kiss on his cheek. Her lips hovering close to his, she whispered, "I anticipated a kiss tonight, but you gave me so much more."

"But not enough?"

She gently poked his chest and said, "If anyone's going to inch his way in, you have the inside track."

Gently swaying her side to side, he teased, "I can do so much with that sloppy phrasing."

Ignoring his silliness, she said, "I need time to—"

"To drive me mad with desire?"

"To trust my own judgment."

He held her close and teased, "A man can only wait so long, so I'll give you 'til your ninety-ninth birthday. Then I need to cut you loose."

"That would make you one hundred and four. You'll need enhancement drugs."

"You enhance me."

Burying her face in his chest, she told him, "I've never felt safe in a man's arms."

He held her tighter, stared at the lights twinkling through a patch of trees below, and said, "When you believe I'm holding you in my head and heart, you'll feel safe in my arms."

Chapter Six

THEY SNUGGLED IN EACH OTHER'S ARMS WATCHING A MOVIE when the buzzer signaled time to pull the fresh apple pie Jenna baked out of the oven. Calling an intermission, Steve shuffled to the refrigerator and grabbed a beer.

"You want one?" he asked, picking at the pie cooling on the wire rack.

"Water, please."

"For my lady," he said, handing her a bottle as he followed her to the couch and plopped down beside her.

She tossed the remote away from him and said lustily, "Your eyes will pop when you see the dress I bought for the Senior Autumn Ball I'm chaperoning next Saturday."

He pulled her across the couch and said, "This body would make a dress made out of recycled refuse look exquisite."

"I need something less biodegradable, something more alive and vibrant to complete my look," she told him, resting her head on his shoulder.

He placed his beer on the coffee table and started to caress her cheek when Jenna's phone rang.

Rolling her eyes, she said, "Sam calls at the most inopportune times."

"For once, don't answer. She has a terminal case of whinorrhea."

"She needs to talk to someone, Steve. I'll make it short."

"Thank God you picked up. I called seven other people, and all's I get are answering machines. No one ever calls back 'cause they're all so busy with their lives. I keep tryin', but it's," she whispered, "so hard."

After all these years, Sam's childish whimpers still sent shivers up Jenna's spine.

"I wish I was with you right now, Jen. You always hug me. I want someone to hug me," she pleaded in a childish voice. After a stream of sniffles, Sam muttered, "Theyneverever huggedme." In a matter-of-fact voice, she told Jenna, "If I cried, my mother'd slap the hell out of me, so I neeever eeever cried." She let out a sarcastic laugh. "My mom enjoyed making me hold her cigarette until the ashes burned down to my fingers. Oooh yeah. I'd screeeam! She'd beat me and beat me and beat me for screaming. I'd scrub and scrub the floors. My father'd come home drunk, wake me up, drag me by my hair to," a hiccup escaped her, "to clean the sink after he peed in it. He forced me to scrub it clean." In between groans she said, "One night, my mom screamed at him fer waking me. She tripped him on the stairs. I grabbed the banister and watched him tumble down and hit his head. Knocked out cold. Pretended he died." With resignation, she said, "He didn't. Maybe they would've loved me if I wasn't such a pig."

"Sam, you're a human sanitizing machine. Something in them was broken. It was never about you. They would've tortured baby Jesus in his manger on Christmas Day if he were their son."

"It sure felt like itwasabout me. So many blackandblue marks. Black and blue all over. Feltlike it was about me."

"No matter how much we try, our love can't fix emotionally ill people. Your mom and dad needed counseling. It wasn't available back then."

"It was too available, so stop defending them," Sam yelled. Child-like she asked, "'Member when Miss Ryan taught us about 'good touches and bad touches'? My mom beat me after I came home and told her we could . . . Why didn't she take me to the shelter?"

"She probably was so afraid and embarrassed to let anyone learn what was happening in your house. She didn't want people to blame her."

"It was her fault. She didn't stop it! She never ever stopped it."

"That's true, but you can't change the past. Now you're free to get the help you need. A good doctor can find the right medication to help you cope with bad memories."

Steve motioned for Jenna to cut the conversation short, but Jenna mouthed, "Fifteen minutes."

He sank into the couch.

"I can't talk for long, Sam. Steve and I are getting ready to—"

"Getting ready to what?" she asked. "Screw?" Her shrill voice reached Steve when she yelled, "I feel like driving there right now. I feel like chopping off his twelve-inch penis with a serratedbutcherknife. I'll rip it off with my teeth! Rip off every pingle senis on everysingleman on every single planet! Earth, Mars, Venus, Jupiter." After a pause, she asked, "Do you think penises are gigantic on Jupiter? Anyway, why can't liquor stores deliver? People wouldn't have to drive drunk when they run out of vodka."

"Stay out of your car when you're drunk, Sam."

Sam laughed carelessly. "Worried 'bout me, or 'bout potherpeople; I mean," she said more distinctly, "other people who have families that love them?"

"Both."

Drained of energy, Sam said, "How 'bout if I take a little, tiny nap first, then go to the store? I never ever wannahurt anyone."

"That's positive thinking. A nap will do you good."

"I love you, Jen."

"I love you, too, Sam."

Fiddling with the phone, Sam mumbled, "I never hear 'Iloveyou' 'cept when you sayit. My motherandfather never said, 'I love you.' How could they? They never even loved each other. I never ever had a birthdayparty, Jen."

"Are you in bed, Sam?"

As Sam struggled to hold the phone, pour more liquor in her glass, and take a sip before she fell into bed, there was a loud crash. Glass shattered on the floor. Panic seizing her, Sam whispered, "Shhh, shhh, shhh. Clean it up! I need to clean it up! Please, please," she said, still whispering, "help me clean it up, Jen." Her voice shaking, she said, "They'll killl meee!"

"It's okay, Sam. They're dead. They can't hurt you anymore."

"You'd think being buried under six feet of dirt would stop them," she whispered, "but believe me, they're always here. Come help me clean, Jen. My junk's safer than Stephen the Demon's junk," she said, giggling at her own joke. Garbling her words, she added, "Let's cutoff hispenis." Between hiccups she said, "If every woman . . . cutoffjust one . . . Men would be extinct. They'd put us on postage stamps."

After several moments of silence, Jenna gently tossed the phone onto the floor and caught Steve's stare from the corner of her eye.

"Come on, Stephen! She's drunk."

Crossing his arms over his chest, he held his stare.

Trying hard not to laugh, Jenna asked, "How do you expect her to feel about men after her father violated her all those years? Give her a chance to get to know you."

"That psychotic woman will never come within a fifty-mile radius of my manhood."

More seriously, she defended Sam saying, "She functions rather well considering the two people who should've loved and protected her betrayed her from the moment of birth."

"There's a reason why people cut her loose, Jenna. She's hopeless."

Saddened by his attitude, she said, "Some chronically stingy people with more than their share of blessings may be just as hopeless." Raising her chin in mild defiance, she asked, "How much more despair would define Mike's life had his family not sacrificed for him? Sam's mother sacrificed Sam." She picked up a pillow, gently whacked him with it, and said, "Penis decapitation seems like a fair punishment for men who leave women so damaged that they're forced to beg for scraps of love and acceptance from strangers. Even if by a miracle, a man falls in love with Sam, she'd be too petrified to enjoy the physical aspect of the relationship."

Raising his hands high over his head in retreat, he said, "You win, but if by some cataclysmic event I'm forced to be under the same roof as Psycho Sam, I'm installing deadbolts on the bedroom door. That decision, my pretty, is non-negotiable."

"Fair enough." With a soft reprimand, she added, "And stop calling her a psycho."

Drinking his beer, he asked, "Do you think she'd really decapitate a man if she had the chance?"

"There's more chance of me slithering into your room and—"

Shooting her a lusty smile, he pulled her close to him, and said, "Show me! Show me your slither."

Palming his chest, she said, "I'd rather talk about how I need to use you—"

"Puhleeze! Use me."

She grabbed his mouth with her fingers and said, "I need an escort to the dance." As she planted a kiss on his mouth, he sucked in her lips, forcing her to pull away to catch her breath.

Resting his head on the back pillow of the couch, he asked, "Am I your last resort?"

Answering sheepishly, she said, "You don't have a lot of free time. I wasn't sure if you'd want to give up an evening for a high school dance." With a slight tilt of her head she said, "I'd like to show you off."

He pulled back, placed his beer on the table, and asked, "Are you the same lady who feared the sight of us together would cause a seismic shift in Spartan Land?"

"At first, I needed to be sure we—"

Raising his hand, he said, "Let's not rehash it." He picked up his beer, took a drink, and bragged, "Wait 'til you see my tux."

"A tux is overkill. Guys generally wear nice suits, and the girls wear evening dresses."

"Bland versus elegant. How sexist is that?"

She lay across his lap, tapped his lips, and said, "Most men hate tuxes."

He held her head an inch away from his face and told her, "I'm wearing my tux."

"Wear a tux if you want. Make it easy for everyone in the banquet room to spot which man is not like the others."

Playing with her, his lips latched onto the side of her neck. Between kisses he said, "How 'bout . . . if I make it easy . . . for kids . . . to pick out which teacher's . . . not like the others?"

"How come everyone I know needs medication?" she cried, wiggling out of his clutch. "Gosh! I swear I never met anyone who delighted in menacing people the way you do."

"I'm wearing my tux," he said with finality. He gulped the rest of his beer, pointed the bottle at her, and said, "Get one more thing straight. I don't dance."

"I can teach you how to dance, Steve." Rolling off his lap, she held out her hands, and said, "Come on."

He shooed her away saying, "Let's not go there. Besides, I'd like to finish this movie before Mike comes home."

She cuddled next to him and asked, "Do you think Mike will mind that we chaperone together?"

He grabbed a handful of peanuts and said, "He already brought it to my attention. I told him if you wanted me there, you would've asked me a long time ago. He seemed disappointed."

Satisfied with herself, she said, "Well, now I've made everyone happy."

He cradled her in his arms and told her, "You can make me happier."

"Give me time to work on that."

The evening of the Autumn Ball was warm and sultry. The rosy-fingered dusk invited romance as Steve pulled up to Jenna's apartment in his white, 1957 Ford Thunderbird. Poised to present her with a single red rose when she opened the door, he stood transfixed on the dazzling beauty that twirled around two times like a ballerina kicking up magic dust all around the room. After slow motioning to a standstill, she asked, "What do you think?"

She didn't have to beg a compliment. Breathless for a moment, he extended his open hand. "This belongs to you."

A miniature, crystal glass slipper sparkled on the palm of his hand. She swooned for a second, then said, "The more I wear it, the better it feels. It's perfect."

Carefully positioning the slipper in a prominent place on her mantle, she touched her nose with the rose and breathed in the sweet fragrance. Reaching for her satin clutch, she turned to inspect him before they left her apartment.

"Where's your tux?"

He tugged gently at one cuff then the other. "Mike insisted I'd feel out of place with tails."

She dragged her hand across her brow. "I guess common sense skipped a generation in the Gaone family."

As they entered the ballroom, Steve marveled at the decorations. Jenna explained, "Every year, we transform this gym into an autumn wonderland. It's like stepping into a fantasy world."

He played with her fingers and said, "I have a fantasy. I dream of—"

Her eyes tripled in size. "Not here," she whispered between clenched teeth. "These kids eavesdrop and misconstrue everything they hear." Issuing a playful reprimand, she said, "If you incite, I'll take you right home and make you go to bed without a snack."

He placed his finger on his lips and said, "Shhhh. These kids will misconstrue what you just said." Quickly scanning the gymnasium, his eyes came around to her. "That sounded tempting."

Nudging him in the side, she was about to counter when Marcus Wright tapped her on the shoulder. Shaking hands with Steve, he said, "Glad you joined us tonight. Did she fill you in on the tradition?"

Steve's eyes swung to Jenna.

Jenna held his hand and said, "It's nothing to worry about. I'll take care of it."

Steve eyed Marcus, "I don't like surprises."

Marcus flashed a bright smile and told Jenna, "I'll help you drag him out on the floor if you have to."

As Marcus walked away to help some students with the stage equipment, Steve straightened his tie, tugged at his cuffs, and asked, "You don't really expect me to dance?"

Growing concerned, she asked, "Why do you have an aversion to dancing?"

His eyes dropped. "After all these years, you'd think I'd get over what they did to me at my high school prom." He raised his chin and looked down at her for several seconds. "But in fairness, the thought of roughing it at my camp makes you uncomfortable, so if I have to muddle through a slow dance, I'll do that for you."

She gently massaged his hand and said, "Camping is different than dancing. You're the only one who'll witness my ineptness in the wilderness." Cupping his cheek with her hand, she said, "I won't let you embarrass yourself in front of these kids." With a sweet smile, she held his hand tighter, and promised, "I'll keep you safe."

Raising his brows, he said, "Still, I wish you would've warned me."

"I tried to, but you said you didn't want me to teach you any steps." She waved her hand. "It's no big deal, Steve. I'll grab one of the other teachers."

She looked across the dance floor at one massive ball of students jumping up and down in unison. Swinging her eyes to him, she said facetiously, "My gosh, if you stand in the middle of those kids and jump up and down with them, they'd crown you *King of Cool.*" Explaining the yearly tradition, she said, "Marcus breaks up that free-for-all and announces that I'm going to show them what real dancing looks like. I grab an unsuspecting chaperone like this," she gently tugged at his arm, "and we dance a few discernible steps while the kids cheer."

Steve surveyed the students in the middle of the dance floor. He made eye contact with Mike and motioned his head toward the stage. Mike inconspicuously wandered over to where Marcus Wright stood and whispered to him. Marcus mounted the stage, grabbed the microphone, and bellowed, "If you guys had to master the concept of dancing for the state test, this school's scores would tumble into the toilet." Motioning with his hands, he said, "Clear that dance floor, and let Miss Rossi and Mr. Gaone show you how it's done."

Mayhem broke out as students jumped up and down cheering. They lined the perimeter of the floor to catch a better view of the show about to unfold. Jenna abruptly turned to Steve and palmed his chest. "Honest!" she whispered nearly out of breath. "This wasn't supposed to happen. Stand here and just let me do it."

An impish grin claimed Steve's lips as his curled index finger motioned for her to follow him onto the dance floor. His gently gyrating hips sent her into mild shock. Quickly gaining composure, she playfully strutted up to him. Together, they dazzled the students with a performance equal to any of the classic dance scenes from vintage movies included in the popular mash-up videos. As Steve skillfully danced in sync with her, twirled her around with artistic ease, and gyrated several more times apart from her, Jenna wondered with pleasure how much more depth there was to this man with whom she was fast falling in love. After the last note, the students brought down the house with thunderous applause.

Slow dancing in his arms during the chaperone dance, she studied his face with admiration. Her lips caressing his ear, she whispered, "You amazed these kids tonight, and I get the feeling you'll always amaze me."

He rested his cheek on hers and felt her soft, curly hair brush against his chin. "You bring out my best talents."

Pulling back, she palmed his chest, and asked, "How many other talents do you have hidden in there, cowboy?"

His lips brushed against her ear. "Stick around for the rest of my life and find out."

Jenna stopped dancing and searched his eyes. Before she could coax him for clarification, Marcus tapped Steve on the shoulder and said, "I need you for a minute. Someone's interested in doing business with you."

Steve blew her a kiss and walked away with a cryptic smile on his face. His heart stayed with her.

Chapter Seven

JENNA LAY CURLED UP ON THE COUCH MUTTERING OBSCENITIES at a student essay when Myra, her childhood friend and college roommate surprised her with a phone call.

"I'm home for a two-day conference. You free for supper tomorrow? It's been so long."

"I'm clearing my schedule," Jenna told her. "We can shop then—"

Myra broke in saying, "Let's buy matching bras and panties in all kinds of colors."

Jenna said, "I'm into body briefers. They're so comfortable."

"Me too! Funny how even our taste in underwear evolved in sync," Myra said, laughing. "I'm staying at the William Penn, Room 200."

Fighting the hotel stay, Jenna said, "My guest room's free. Stay with me."

"The company's making us stay with teams, so I'm stuck here. Otherwise, I'd like nothing better than to pull an all-nighter with you."

"Wait 'til you hear the latest about Steve," Jen told her.

"Oh, my God, Jen. It must be love."

"No details on the phone, but I will say this: He's so . . ." She purposely let her thought hang.

"He's so what?" Myra asked. "Messing with my imagination constitutes abuse."

"Think of it as payback for what you did to me last year with that Rob, *I-can't-keep-my-hands-off-my-own-genitalia,* Rodgers."

"Good God! Don't remind me of that pathetic specimen. If he hadn't hit on you, I'd be married to a creep."

"Creep's too kind. The pervert had an accomplishment to match every letter of the alphabet, and I let him get up to 'P' . . . as in 'I have a penis as large as the Arabian Peninsula' before I booted him out."

"Being late that day wasn't my fault, Jen." Still somewhat amazed at the turn of events, she let out an incredulous laugh. "Who knew that a lunatic shooting at storefront mannequins up and down Fifth Avenue would cause a lockdown of the whole block and save me from marrying a pervert?"

"I'm glad the crisis worked out for you, and I'm doubly glad you believed me."

"There's not a man alive I'd believe over you, Jen." As the seminar participants reconvened in the conference hall, Myra sounded harried. "My break's over; gotta run. See you tomorrow at four."

When Jenna arrived at the William Penn, she spotted Myra waiting in the lobby. Myra grabbed Jenna, swayed back and forth several times with her, and said, "Come on. I reserved a table in the dining room so we don't have to waste another minute. The first thing you're going to do is update me on Steve."

"It's been a long time since I've fallen for any man as hard as I've fallen for this guy," Jenna confided.

"Does he make your heart pound harder than Ronan King?"

Jenna looked down and massaged her coffee mug.

Myra winced. "I'm sorry, Jen. One of these days I'll learn never to mention the hog's name." With a smirk, she said, "Word is he hasn't changed a bit."

Jenna smiled. The years never seemed to lessen the contempt Myra held for Ronan. How much more indignant would she be toward him if she knew the full fallout from that love affair, Jenna thought.

"Does anyone know what he's doing now?" Jenna asked.

"He's a rising star in New York politics. Rumor has it that he openly cheated on his trophy wife, forced several mistresses to have abortions, and his wife finally bolted without a single penny for her pain and suffering."

Jenna's face blanched.

"Sounds like he hates himself more than he hates women." Myra added, "All he does is ruin lives."

Jenna nodded. "Sometimes I wonder what he would've been like if . . ." Her voice trailed off.

"For starters," Myra said, breaking off a piece of bread, "he wouldn't have desecrated a poetic name." Her eyes widened. "I used to swoon each time the name *Ronan* rolled off our tongues." She squinted and said with eerie intonation, "Now, Judas has a more pleasant sound."

Laughing at her friend's animation, Jenna asked, "You don't really believe a man's name influences his character, do you?"

Myra shrugged. "Who knows what goes on in parents' heads when they name a kid? I know a lady who named her son Angus because she liked cows." She popped a small chunk of bread into her mouth and said between chews, "That's abuse. Still, a cow name is better than a pig name. But to answer your original question, if Ronan would've been married to you, people would've respected him." She dabbed her mouth with a napkin and said, "He did you a favor, Jen. Some guys don't know how to be happy with a good woman. They're like grimy, matted cats that prowl back alleys for any piece of garbage they can find." More seriously, she said, "Ronan has the distinction of leaving life shitty everywhere he goes because he's a first-class asshole." Sipping her water, she said, "That's the difference between Steve and Ronan King. Steve doesn't have to conquer vaginas to prove he's a man. Money and sex don't define him; good character does." Myra wiped the condensation from her glass. "The fact that he's a responsible, single parent speaks volumes."

Jenna forced a smile, sipped her drink, and said, "I hope my warts don't drive him away."

Myra's eyes grew large. "What warts? You're a gem. And you're not just any gem. You're a diamond that outshines and outlasts every other stone." She let out a short laugh. "Who else in this universe still answers the phone when that cuckoo that escaped from the clock calls and harangues for hours?" Myra stared at Jenna and asked, "How is Sam, anyway?"

"Nothing's new. Most of the time she obsesses over her childhood." Jenna played with her napkin and said, "At least she's seeing an analyst, but from the stories she tells me, the doctor seems to be as disturbed as Sam." Rolling her eyes, Jenna asked, "What doctor in her right mind gives an emotionally disturbed patient her private cell number? Sam's emergencies are closer than contractions a half hour before giving birth."

Awestruck, Myra countered, "You should know. She has your number on speed dial. According to you, she's hitting rock bottom every six months." With a wave of her hand, she said, "Believe me, Sam's in better shape than she lets on."

"I don't know, Myra. No normal person whimpers like a child one minute then threatens to cut off a man's penis the next."

Dumbfounded, Myra asked, "Are we talking about the same demented woman who went berserk at the ball game when she mistook that dripping footlong hotdog for a heat-seeking love missile?"

Chuckling, Jenna said, "Gosh, don't remind me. I thought that guy was going to knock her out."

Myra laughed. "I wanted to stuff that footlong down her throat myself, but I didn't want to be responsible for a major psychotic break."

Fighting to catch their breaths from robust laughter, Myra asked, "How could three inches of an all-beef wiener hanging over a toasted bun be responsible for an earth-shattering emotional disturbance in a human being? Sam's bulging eyes made that guy ask her if she wanted a bite. Who knew she'd knock the hotdog out of his hands and let out that blood-curdling scream?"

Their laughter subsiding, Myra played with her napkin and said, "I don't think Sam will be decapitating penises any time soon." She sipped her drink and added, "Still, you're a saint for sticking with her all these years. No more for me. I can understand the footlong fiasco, but when we drove for half the morning and stood on her doorstep and she refused to let us in until we deloused ourselves in that god-awful spray before we could grace her sterile cocoon, that was enough for me. Her house was so damn immaculate you could separate Siamese twins conjoined at the head on her kitchen floor without threat of infection. But of course, there was no meal, because cooking would leave traces of humanity." She reminded Jenna, "The reason why Sam's still alive is because you wouldn't let me grab her neck and squeeze the life out of her after she called me a pig."

Jenna pulled her hair back and laughed until her stomach ached. "She probably popped a nitroglycerin pill when she discovered the wrapper from the candy bar we devoured in the bathroom."

Her palms facing Jenna, Myra said, "I'll do anything for you, Jen, but don't ever ask me to help Sam again unless you're checking her into a psych ward. Mark my words: She's manipulative and certifiable. Who knows how her parents really died? What's to stop her from doing it again?"

"Don't be so hard on her, Myra. No one wants to admit that people turned a blind eye every single day she lived through that torture."

"You believe everything she tells you, Jen, but think about it. She had fantastic friends. We wanted her to room with us in college. She could've received grants because her parents were dead, but I'm still paying off my college loans. I swear she orchestrates misery just so she can perpetuate this 'poor me' life she refuses to abandon. She drives everyone away by talking incessantly about her childhood. What were we supposed to do? We were kids." She sipped her drink and said, "I refuse to enable her distorted, miserable view of life. She clings to *you* because you have a bleeding heart."

Jenna stirred her drink and countered, "We all have families and friends to lean on when we're hurt and afraid. Who does Sam have?"

"She had all of us, but she drove us away. A friendship's give and take. All Sam does is take. She takes up time; she takes up energy, and she refuses to entertain the thought that someone besides her may be experiencing a rough patch in his or her life. She's like an infant who thinks the world ends at her fingertips and toes."

A smile claimed Jenna's face as she folded her napkin and neatly placed it to the side of her plate. Her sympathetic eyes mirrored her sincerity when she said, "Everyone needs someone to help keep the water outta the ship, Myra. Sam has me, and I have you, which means Sam has you, too."

Myra sighed. "Maybe." She rolled a piece of her paper napkin into a ball and flicked it at Jenna. "Can we puhleeze forget Sam for one evening? I'm surprised she hasn't been hounding you as we speak. Tell me some Stephen stories." With enthusiasm, she said, "Good vibes surround him, Jen. If he has any brothers, I'll gouge out the eyes of anyone who tries to grab the bouquet from me at your wedding."

Jenna pulled back, let out a laugh, and asked, "Aren't we a bit premature?"

"Oooh, there's going to be a wedding," Myra predicted, rubbing her palms together. "I feel it in my bones."

Jenna's eyes rolled. "More like early onset of arthritis."

Myra pointed and teased, "Mark my words. I'm dining with the future Mrs. Gaone."

Jenna told Myra one Stephen story after another until the restaurant emptied. Caught up on each other's lives, they mourned the evening's end.

"We never shopped for underwear, Jen."

"No one sees our underwear anyway," Jenna said, shrugging.

"Gotta give that guy of yours credit for trying," Myra countered.

Dragging out their goodbyes, they carried their conversation to the lobby of the hotel. Jenna promised, "I'll call once a month to let you know I'm alive."

"You take the even months; I'll take the odd," Myra suggested before hopping on the elevator to her room.

Jenna slipped into her car where memories washed over her. A nauseous feeling crept in as losses lingered: Josh, Ronan, and the part of herself she kept hidden from the people she loved.

Chapter Eight

A DUSTING OF SNOW SETTLED ON SPARTA EARLY FRIDAY morning and vanished in the warm, mid-day sun. The early November snowfall served as a reminder that blustery cold winds were not far behind. Procrastinators of unfinished summer recreation would have to hurry or forfeit the pleasures until the distant spring.

With time to spare after a late afternoon meeting, Steve swung by Jenna's apartment and said, "I can use some help this weekend preparing the cabin for winter. You in?"

Intending to be seductive, she twisted her hair around her index finger and teased, "I'm not the camping type, but with this much effort," she held her thumb and index finger close together, "I bet you can talk me into a weekend at the Waldorf."

He gently palmed the back of her neck, pulled her close, and kissed her forehead. "It'll be you, me, and nature. You'll never choose blinking neon signs and loud horns honking in a congested city over my slice of heaven again."

Anchored in growing familiarity, she sat on the couch, tucked her legs underneath her, and asked, "How can you possibly have fun with a woman who cringes at the sight of critters that crawl, barfs at the suggestion of roasting rabbits, and," she emphasized the word, "refuses to skinny-dip in a lake with slithering snakes and snapping turtles?"

"It's called desperation, Rossi. I need someone to help me chop and stack wood. Mike needs to make practice Saturday morning; my brother's out of town." He kissed her hard on the lips. "I'm stuck with you." He stood, looked down at her, and said, "Besides, you're the lady who bragged about how rugged you are." He raised his hands to both sides of his head and fashioned bull horns. "You're the lady bull rider." He grabbed her hands and pulled her up into his arms. "Lend me some of that brawn this weekend." Without waiting for an answer, he looked at his watch and pecked her on the cheek. "We'll leave right after the game. Pack light."

The night air was cold and crisp when they pulled up to the cabin porch. Shivering, Jenna clung to her jacket while Steve lugged several logs to the fireplace and coaxed a small fire. Gradually, a steady blaze warmed the room. He unpacked the truck as she claimed the ottoman positioned a few feet from the flaming logs and pondered how comfortable their relationship had grown in such a brief time. Although he avoided using the word love, the way he looked at her, the way he touched her, the way he afforded her every consideration radiated his depth of feeling for her. Despite her unspoken love for him, she had no intention of breaking a promise she made to herself that day long ago in the convent in France. Any relationship worth offering up her body and soul had to be grounded in a formal commitment.

I owe him the truth, she thought, but not tonight. I can't bear to watch him walk away in this beautiful place.

"Sleep in whatever room you want, but don't come waltzing into my room all hours of the night when Smokey smells his next meal."

She shot him a sideways glance. "Smokey?"

"A hungry black bear that's been foraging around the cabins. He has a taste for soft, sensuous, human, female flesh. He's been off the radar for a couple of weeks, so he's either dead or more likely famished."

She unbuttoned her jacket and let it drop to the floor. She pulled back her hair, offered a nervous laugh, and feigned calm. "Don't try to scare me into your bed, cowboy."

Wondering how long she'd be able to deflect his overtures for intimacy, she tested his resolve by asking, "Why don't you just ask me to sleep with you? I can say 'no' for the umpteenth time in my life because I need a . . ." She looked up at him with unsure eyes, then quickly turned her gaze to the fire. "Maybe if I'm lucky, Smokey will end my misery."

Her eyes followed him moving from one room to the other, readying the kitchen and stacking the cupboards with non-perishable goods. Projecting on him the feeling that he had buyer's remorse, she pushed harder to elicit a response.

"You would've had a better time inviting a bimbo to camp with you instead of a Victorian prude." Crossing her arms, she stared at the flickering flames and braced herself for his response.

He finished stacking several cases of water on the counter and wiped the sink clean. A fly, late for dormancy, lighted on his clean counter, causing him to mumble a curse word before he swatted it. After placing one oil lamp on the kitchen table and one in each bedroom, he wiped his hands clean. Quietly strolling up behind her, he straddled her on the ottoman, and pulled her back to his chest, nestling her close. With exaggerated force, he buried his face in her hair and breathed in the sweet fragrance of brown sugar and figs.

"Is the pretty lady done pouting?"

Sweeping his face through her hair one more time, he told her, "I love the smell of you!" He kissed the back of her neck and said, "I will never use fear to coax you to my bed." Pulling her closer, he said, "And I will never invite a bimbo to share my life. I appreciate intellectual stimulation as well as other forms of stimulation."

The room was quiet except for an occasional creaking of the cabin joints and the crackling logs on the fire. He gently massaged her neck for several seconds then lowered his hands to her shoulders. His fingers moved up and down several times on either side of her spine, gently kneading her muscles like dough before he slid one hand to the front of her. He caressed her stomach then glided up to her chest. She arched her back, but he was ready and pulled her toward him, feeling the softness of her as he planted kisses on her cheek below her ear.

She bent her head back and let out a deep sigh. "Your touch electrifies every fiber in my body. If you're not careful, I'll explode in your arms."

He let out a soft groan, turned her head, and kissed her hard on her mouth. "Save the explosion for this."

His hand slipped down low and caused fear to duel with desire. Fear won out. She slid forward off the ottoman and turned to survey the disappointment on his face. Kneeling before him, she placed her hands on his muscular thighs and consoled him one more time.

"It's not you, Steve. I'm just not ready to go there." Frustrated with herself, she raised her hands in the air, and said, "Maybe I'll never be ready."

He covered his face with his hands for a second, then pushed himself off the stool and playfully rolled on top of her. Gently pinning her beneath him, he pleaded, "Talk to me, Jenna." He held her face in his hands and planted a long, lingering kiss on her lips. "Trust me." Her silence prompted his lips to grab her lips one more time before he did a slow push-up and lifted himself off her. He reached for her hand and pulled her to her feet. Sighing, he said, "Some rest will do us both good. Plan to work every muscle in that beautiful body beginning at dawn."

The aroma of coffee brewing on the wood burner stove woke her early to a dark, lifeless room. As she pulled open the wooden shutters, she blinked her eyes open to a stream of sunlight that shimmered across the floor. Steve looked up from his plate as she slowly shuffled into the kitchen rubbing the sleep from her eyes. Pulling up a chair for her, he sat across the table and watched her cover a wide, long yawn.

With a gruff voice, he teased, "I must've missed the hearse that dropped you off."

Scratching her head with one hand, she pointed to the coffee pot with the other. "A cup of that will resurrect me."

He filled her mug to the rim and passed a plate of bacon and eggs to her. Wiping his mouth with a napkin, he said, "Do what prima donnas do in the wild. When you're ready, join me by the woodpile."

Before he opened the door, she asked, "Is a shower out of the question?"

He turned and said, "The lake's at your disposal." Letting out a laugh, he added, "Don't bother with make-up either. Gloves will protect your nails."

She picked up a strip of bacon with her fingers and said between bites, "Yum, this tastes so good."

"Eat up, diva. No more food 'til five."

"Why so late?" she wanted to know. "Don't mountain folk break for lunch?"

"We'll eat when the work's done."

"You know," she said, raising her chin in the air. "There are easier ways to get rid of me."

He opened the door, turned, and said, "You're as necessary as clean air, fresh water, and plenty of sunshine."

Masking her pounding heart, she bent her head back, and asked, "How many women have fallen for that sweet line?"

"I've only applied it to you."

Biting into another piece of bacon, she slowly surveyed the cabin before fixing her eyes on him. "It seems I underestimated the merits of camping with you."

Holding her gaze, he said, "You underestimate a lot about me."

The early morning November sun was unusually hot, but an intermittent, cool breeze refreshed them as she worked steadily stacking the wood Steve chopped. True to his word, after several hours of intense, non-stop work, he finally rested on a stump and traded his ax for a bottle of water. Downing half the bottle in several gulps, he eyed Jenna, wiped the sweat from his brow with his shirt, and tossed it aside.

"I have to admit, you work like a man."

Shooting him a haughty, wide-eyed stare, she said, "Aren't you the chauvinistic male wonder?"

Chugging more water, he said, "Learn how to accept a compliment, Rossi."

Feeling as though she just stepped out of a sauna, she unzipped her red vest and dabbed the sweat from her face with the bottom edge of her jersey before saying, "I'll make you a deal, Gaone." Her voice was assertive as she pointed her bottle of water at him and said, "When you learn how to give a lady a compliment, I'll find it easier to accept a compliment."

Carrying a smug look, she guzzled more water, wiped her mouth with the back of her hand, and screwed on the cap. In the second it took for her to turn to stack more wood, he leaped on her like a puma pounces on its prey. He grabbed one of her shapely arms and pulled her hard up against his bare chest. Her surprise wore off quickly, as his perspiration bled through her floral print jersey.

Meeting her eyes squarely, he said, "You're the smartest, prettiest woman I've ever made break a sweat." He planted a hard kiss on her lips and said, "How about if I cool this hot body off?" Running his hands sensuously over her breasts and moving around down her back, he hoisted her off the ground, and said, "In the lake!"

Her scream was short, as if he squeezed all the breath out of her. Stuttering protests, she kicked and tugged to free herself from his stronghold.

"No, Steve! Put me down!" Flailing her arms, she thrust her body back and forth like a ten-pound catfish hooked on one of his lines. She kicked until she felt the ground beneath her feet. He playfully continued to pull her toward the lake as she threatened, "If you throw me in, I'll walk home. I'll never come back. Never!"

He picked her up, pressed her against him, pushed his face into her chest for several seconds, and gently let her body slide along his until her feet touched the ground. He locked eyes with her and whispered, "Do you have any idea how much I love being with you?"

Her breath came back slow and easy. A soft smile crossed her lips as she draped one arm around his neck and with her free hand played with the wet hairs on his chest. "Half as much as I love being with you?"

His lips grabbed her mouth causing sensation to mount in him. His desire for her was overwhelming, but he knew she'd resist. Kissing her hard one more time, he broke away. She watched him jog down to the dock like he was a wild man engulfed in flames. He kicked off his shoes and plunged into the lake. A loud, "Ahhh," hung in the air as he disappeared into the depths.

She flew up the path to the cabin and grabbed a towel, his sweatpants, and the blanket still sprawled in front of the hearth from the night before.

"Did you jump into this freezing lake to save my honor?" she asked, stifling laughter as he wrestled with his wet jeans. She draped the blanket over his shoulders as he pulled on his dry, warm sweats.

He shivered for several moments until the sun beating down on the blanket and her fingers massaging his back generated warmth through him. He pointed at her and said, "Next time, you're going in!" Holding the edges of the blanket under his chin, he jutted his jaw and surveyed the lake. "I may as well catch some fish while I'm wet and the sun's still warm." Tossing the blanket off to the side, he rolled his shoulders to relax his muscles and said, "We worked through lunch, so let's cook an early dinner." Eyeing her, he said, "Bait the hooks."

Raising her brows in casual surprise, she asked, "You expect me to pierce a live crayfish with a metal hook and call that fun?"

"Fun's secondary when you have to eat, Jenna. Hand me the bait."

With an uppity voice, she badgered, "If you would've stopped at a restaurant along the way, we could've bought barbecued chicken and potato salad. We'd be feasting right now instead of killing helpless animals."

"Let's deal with what we have." Pointing to the cabin, he said, "Get the crayfish and hand them to me."

She jogged up to the porch, found the bait and pole, and lugged them back down to the dock. Handing him the pole, she said, "I'll eat crackers and peanut butter. I don't want to kill any fish."

After grappling with a crayfish, he pierced it with the hook, cast the line far out into the lake, then turned to her and asked, "Why is it that catching, cooking, and eating fresh fish rankles you, but picking up a bucket of barbecued chicken at a diner doesn't mar your sensibilities? I noticed that piercing a sharp steak knife into filet mignon and scarfing down lobster tails at every restaurant we frequent doesn't cause any emotional damage either."

Offering weak absolution for herself, she countered, "For starters, I'm not the one killing the animal."

"So, if a middle man does your dirty work, it's acceptable to feast on the flesh of innocent animals?"

Rolling her eyes, she said, "I can tell it bothers you that I don't like killing animals."

"Not wanting to kill animals is understandable. What's baffling is your unwillingness to fight with equal ferocity to stop the slaughter of sad-eyed cows, little piglets, and those cute little lambs as you do a dumb fish in this lake."

Sitting beside him on the dock with their feet dangling close to the surface of the water, she asked, "Are you done?"

Before he could answer, a heavy tug on the line caught him off guard. He instinctively began to reel in the largemouth bass struggling to free itself.

He yelled, "Grab the net!"

Jumping around, she screamed, "Oh my gosh! Look at that thing wiggling and thrashing." She knelt down close behind him, shoved him forward several times, and said, "Let it go, Steve. Don't kill it."

Shrugging her off at the same time he reeled in the fish and grabbed the net himself, he yelled, "Calm down, Jenna, or you'll be swimming with all the other largemouths you're so eager to save." Shaking his head at her juvenile behavior, he suggested, "If you can't stop flopping around like your friend here, make yourself useful and light the fire. Let me catch a couple more, and supper will be ready."

Feigning insult, she asked, "Did you just threaten me?"

His look dared her to linger one second longer before he grabbed hold of her ankle and said, "The first chance I get, you're going in."

She wiggled loose, looked down at him, and laughed. "How am I supposed to feel comfortable in the wilderness with a man who keeps threatening me?"

He cocked his head, closed one eye, and said, "And she's still standing on this dock."

She gave his earlobe a gentle tug and said, "I'll ignore that third threat, but meditate on this while I go start the fire. If you can kill a helpless fish, an innocent rabbit, or a graceful deer, you're one step closer to killing a human being."

He cast the line hard and long before turning to her and saying, "Be still for five seconds and tell me from where you manage to gather all this psycho analytical babble you're spewing. Do you think Adolph Hitler was an avid fisherman? The deranged bastard probably never thought of harming a rabbit or squirrel in his life, but he sure as hell had no qualms about murdering millions of innocent human beings." Tilting his head, he said seductively, "If you want to make up for all this needless drama, babe, all you have to do is light my fire."

Kneeling behind him, she gently ran her fingertips up and down his bare back, and said, "I just don't like watching animals die."

He leaned back on her, turned his head to face her, and said convincingly, "Then you need to become a vegan." With an impish glint in his eye, he continued saying, "Right now, you can light my—"

"You think that phrase is clever, don't you?"

"All I'm saying is you're the only woman who holds the power to light the fire to end my hunger."

The autumn morning sun warmed her skin as she leisurely leaned back against the porch post to soak up the beauty of the placid lake. Several birds soared high in the sky as her eyes rolled over the partially bare garden where a lone bee fumbled the hardy mums. Frightened chipmunks scurried to safety. Beneath the dark, bare-branched trees swaying elegantly against the bright blue sky, a row of mallards quickly filed into the lake as the truck door slammed shut scaring them off. Her eyes swung toward the stone walkway where leaves floated down the path that intersected the gravel road leading back to the city. As Steve loaded the last cooler on the truck, he poked fun saying, "Let's get you back to Insanity Land before irreparable damage takes hold."

A cold current ran through her as she fixed her eyes on him tugging at a rope that he used to tie down a tarp that covered some tools. Wrapping her arms around her legs, she sat motionless as pools threatened to overflow onto her cheeks. He turned and read the anguish on her face.

She looked away.

Running his hand through his hair, he bounded past the three stairs, straddled her from behind, and locked her in his arms tightening his squeeze.

"I'm not letting you go until we settle this right now."

Shivering under the warm sun, she said, "You'll let me go as soon as . . ." Her voice trailed off.

"As soon as what?" he asked, giving her a quick shake.

She held tight to the back of his hand pressing on her chest. After several moments of silence, she told him, "His name was Ronan King." Unable to turn and meet his eyes, she stared at the far-off horizon and said, "I was a stupid freshman who followed him around like one of those puppies you talk about." Wiping her wet cheeks with her hands, she told him, "I thought he loved me as much as I loved him." Letting out a sarcastic laugh, she added, "He told me I was the only girl he invited to his frat house. When he was done, he zipped up his pants and said, 'Get dressed. You need to get outta here.'" She took a deep breath and let out a heavy sigh. "I felt so dirty, so cheap." She pulled her hair over her shoulder and leaned back as if relieved to unburden her heart with the secret she carried for almost half her life. "He couldn't get me into his bed fast enough, but he shoved me out even faster."

Resting his chin on her shoulder, he watched the rise and fall of her chest.

She broke the silence saying, "I've spent the rest of my life trying to forget." Drying her face with her hands again, she turned to him, and said, "I'm afraid to trust my heart. Love hurts too much." She turned away and stared at the ground.

He buried his face in her hair and whispered, "Love doesn't hurt, Jenna. What you experienced with *Ronan*," he exaggerated the name, "wasn't love."

She took a deep breath and exhaled slowly. Standing, she faced him and blinked back fresh tears. He reached for her hand, but she shook her head, crossed her arms, and held them tightly over her chest to confine her shame.

"You made love; he had sex."

Her eyes dropped.

"Look at me, Jen."

Raising her eyes, she stared at him with guilty defiance.

"You fell for the wrong guy. Now you're with the right guy." After a slight pause, he added, "Unless your heart's still with him."

Before she looked away, her eyes revealed a deeper connection to Ronan that her silence failed to mask.

Steeling himself for the possibility of losing her, he asked, "Do you still love him?"

Her eyes darted to his. Giving her head one, hard shake, she looked off to the side and said with soft remorse, "I had his baby." Swinging her eyes back to him, she said, "When I found out I was pregnant, I begged my parents to let me study abroad for a year. I gave birth to a little girl in France but didn't tell my parents until months after the delivery and adoption."

Her heart sagged as she watched Steve sit expressionless. She looked away focusing her glacial stare on the bare trees in the distance. With little emotion, she told him, "The Mother Superior helped me give my baby away to an American couple living on the outskirts of Paris for a year." Her eyes dropped as she gently kicked some stones. "Every Friday at supper time, I'd make a pilgrimage to a convent in the valley where I'd say a prayer in the most serene chapel. The Mother Superior guessed I was pregnant. She begged me to involve my parents," a sarcastic laugh escaped her, "but you know me. I'm the lady with all the answers."

A silent gulf separated them as a cool breeze rustled some dried leaves caught in one of the corners of the porch. Steve leaned back, propping himself up on his elbows.

"How did *Ronan*," he exaggerated the name again, "react?"

"He doesn't know. I didn't want to face more rejection." Glancing at him sideways, she searched his face for some sign of emotion, but he only sat and stared at her. She ended saying, "You deserve more than a hermit crab who's been hiding in a better shell than her own." Her back to him, she could feel him watching her as she scanned the peaceful lake. Turning to face him, she held his gaze for several moments before saying, "I won't bind you to any sweet promises you've lavished on me for the past months. You were talking to an imposter." Looking down, she walked halfway to the truck then hesitated. Turning, she said, "You're the only one besides my mother and father I trust with the truth about what happened in France that year."

He leaned against the porch post as a barrage of thoughts tumbled through his mind. What would life be like without Michael? Who would have read him stories? Would he have crawled into another man's bed during the thunder storms? Would he be high-fiving another guy after a good game? His eyes settled on Jenna leaning on the back of the truck resting her head on her forearms.

"My brother, Phil, can help us find her."

Jenna looked up. "It's too late. She has a family, and I'll never be a part of it." She let out a self-deprecating laugh. "I buy Christmas ornaments every year that remind me of her. I've fabricated this elaborate pipe dream where we decorate the tree together, drink hot cocoa, and share family stories, but I know in the end she's not mine, and I'll never hold her in my arms again."

"Do you want to be a part of her life?"

She pulled her hair back over one shoulder. "I don't want to convolute her life any more than I already have. I'm not even sure the adoption was legal."

He stood and drew her into his arms. She rested her head on his chest and turned her eyes to peer out over the lake where ducks were comically dipping their heads in and out of the water, flapping their wings, and skimming the surface of the pond. She buried her face deeper into his chest and pleaded, "Right now, I'll settle for you not hating me."

He held her at arm's length, gave her a stern look, and said, "You've never settled for anything in your life. Why start now?" Drawing her back into his arms, he whispered, "We'll get through this."

After several seconds of silence, she said, "I didn't love my baby the way you loved yours."

Guiding her to the porch, he sat and patted the space next to him. "There's no shortage of fraudulence, Jenna." Following a hawk soaring across the sky, he said, "To this day my parents don't know Amy threatened to have an abortion." When Jenna's eyes widened, he asked, "Amazing, huh? My mother would've used both of us for fish bait if I let that happen." Looking out over the lake, he admitted, "Hell, I spent the first three years of Mike's life being jealous of all the attention my mother showered on him." Covering his face with his hands, he gave voice to something he had been ashamed to acknowledge for so long. "My mother and I are at odds because I don't know how to express gratitude. The truth is I'll never be able to express my appreciation for her sacrifices, so I minimize her help. I'm convinced she knows why I'm doing it." He draped his arm over Jenna's shoulders and pulled her close. "I jumped out of the nest and crash landed. She picked me up, dusted me off, and kept chewing my food for me until I got strong and developed wings." He snapped the stem of a late blooming mum growing near the porch steps and handed it to her. "You grew up faster than I ever did." His lips grazed her hand as he said, "It took courage to love your child enough to lose her rather than chance the King family ruining her life. That's the kind of selfless, unconditional love every child deserves."

Hooking his arm around her waist, he led her to the truck. He lifted his chin and said, "I found out something important about you today."

That's an understatement, she thought as she dabbed the corners of her eyes with a tissue.

"Think about it. We both chose life for our kids even though we believed our lives were ruined."

With mild awe, she lifted his hand to her lips, kissed it, and said, "This is the first time I've thought about my baby without hating myself for giving her away. I can't stop missing her."

His brows rose.

She stopped and asked, "Does missing her surprise you?"

"Not at all. You just opened the possibility of why the French never say, 'I miss you.'"

"French people miss their loved ones like everyone else," she told him.

"Of course, they do, but their phrasing captures the essence of being apart better than other languages. They say, '*Tu me manques*,' which means, 'You are missing from me.' It's a more painful separation, a fragmentation, like a missing part of a body. It's the way you miss your baby." Reflecting more personally, he added, "It's the way I'd feel if I lost you."

As they drove down the dirt road, he said, "One thing really confuses me about your story, Jen."

Her stomach churned, fearful that this one small tug at her veracity would unravel the whole love affair.

"I can't put a positive spin on the fact that the name," he exaggerated "*Ronan*, didn't make you run for the hills." He muttered, "Ronan's one helluvah ugly little rich kid's name."

"My gosh," she said, relieved by his casual demeanor, "Myra hates his name, too. Ronan's a nice name; he just wasn't a nice person."

Staring straight ahead, he asked, "In all your years of teaching, what's the classiest boy's name you've encountered?"

She pretended to ponder for several seconds before saying, "Michael's definitely a solid name."

"We're past pandering, Miss Rossi."

Eyeing him as he skillfully maneuvered past several potholes in the dirt road, she countered, "I'm doing no such thing. Stop playing Rumplestiltskin, forcing me to come up with a preconceived name." She clasped her fingers between his and squeezed. "How about Holstein?"

Narrowing his eyes, he said, "Only if you give birth to a side of beef."

"You're right," she told him. "Better to give birth to a martyr and name him *Stephen,*" she exaggerated the name.

"Give the pretty lady a cigar!" he said with bravado. "At least we're not perverts preying on people who love us."

With worry in her voice, she said, "I don't blame you for disliking Ronan, but promise me if you ever run into him on business, you'll walk away."

His face tightened.

"Promise me," she pleaded.

He stared dead ahead, cranked up the volume to the CD player, and said, "I really like this song."

Chapter Nine

TWO WEEKS BEFORE THANKSGIVING, CLARE GAONE CALLED Steve and said, "I need to borrow your deep fryer to cook the turkey."

"I'll drop it off on my way to the office."

"Since when do you work on Sunday? I'm on my way to Aunt Mary's. I'll stop by and share a hot cup of tea with you."

"It's the only day my client can meet, but come on over. I'll spare a couple of minutes for the lady who changed my diapers."

"You had the cutest and cleanest bum on the East Coast. Even your dirtiest diapers never caused a stink."

Rolling his eyes, he said, "I'll add that to my resume."

"I'm on my way, smarty pants."

Clare sat at Steve's kitchen table, her eyes following him around the room. He handed his mother a mug, dropped a teabag in it, then poured hot water to start the brew.

"I ran into Jenna in the mall a couple of days ago," Clare told him. "She's all excited about inviting you to Thanksgiving dinner at her mother's house, so I invited her to stop by our house." She picked on a chocolate doughnut and added, "That girl's an absolute doll. Her whole family's wonderful."

Offering a packet of sugar to Clare, Steve said, "Jenna told me you two talked. So why the special trip to tell me again?"

Stirring the sugar into the tea, she told him, "I thought I'd pick up the roaster and spend some quality time talking with you."

"Purge it, Mom. Then we can move on with our lives."

Popping the rest of the doughnut into her mouth and chewing as she talked, she said, "I really like Jenna." Dabbing her mouth with a napkin, she added, "Too bad you didn't marry someone like her in the first place."

"Where would I be without Mike? Where would you be without Mike?" Grabbing a bottle of water from the refrigerator, he turned to her and cautioned, "Don't let him hear you say that. Amy loved him, and he loved his mother every bit as much as I love you."

Deadpanned, she said, "I may be opinionated, but I'm not insensitive."

She slipped her purse onto her shoulder and stood to leave. Her hand on the doorknob, she turned and said, "Even though I don't like some of your choices, we've always been proud of the way you and Phil turned out."

Pressing his fingers on his eyelids, he said, "Can't you just once give a compliment without slipping in the dig?"

"What dig? You don't have to like every choice someone makes to be proud of him." Fumbling for her keys, she said, "Not to change the subject, but make sure you get to the house before the Thanksgiving circle."

His eyes narrowed. "Is that the reason you're bonding with me this morning?"

"Goodness, Stephen. You've been seeing Jenna for months. Don't you think it's time to introduce her to your aunts and uncles?"

"You want the truth? I cringe at the thought of everyone being thankful that I finally found a nice woman. Then I have to brace myself for some relative who will compare Jenna to Amy and talk about how I almost messed up my life." After several gulps of water, he said, "Not only is it embarrassing, Mike's not stupid. He knows how the family feels about his mother."

Clare cupped Steve's cheek and said, "Do you know, for the longest time, no matter how successful you'd become, I laid awake nights worrying about you?" Light mist blanketed her eyes. "Your father maintains that for the last eighteen years I've been in a constant state of turmoil over you." She ran her index finger under her eye and said, "I don't care what people say. You were always a nice kid, and you deserve happiness. You deserve a good woman who loves you," she let out a short laugh, "almost as much as I love you." Standing straight and pretending to be stoic, she raised her hand high and swore an oath. "Invite Jenna to Thanksgiving dinner." She dragged her thumb and index finger across her lips. "I'll zip it."

Smirking, he said, "Sure you will. And we'll all bow down to the East when the evangelicals adopt Sharia Law."

Lugging the cumbersome fryer to his mother's car, Steve made her a proposition. "Don't embarrass me on Thanksgiving Day, and I'll foot the bill for a weekend in Vegas."

Being silly, she said, "I know why you picked Vegas, Stephen."

"Only one reason, Mom. Your honeymoon suite's in Vegas."

"You think 'What happens in Vegas stays in Vegas.' Well life's not Vegas, but I'll still take the deal."

With one eye closed, he philosophized, "Life's a lot like Vegas, Mom. Sometimes you win; sometimes you lose, but most of the time the deck's stacked against you."

Surprised, she countered, "Why so pessimistic, sweetie? Despite the odds, you made a nice life for Amy, Mike, and yourself. Odds are you'll make an even nicer life with Jenna."

"Slow down, Mom." With an air of futility, he said, "I've only known the lady for several months. Don't talk marriage in front of Mike or the family. Let me broach that topic if that time comes."

"Stop worrying, Stephen. I'm telling *you* how I feel. I'm not broadcasting our business to the world."

As he watched his mother drive away, he thought, I can't live with or without that woman.

Despite the lingering sensation of the foodgasm they experienced earlier at the Rossi dinner, Jenna and Steve were excited to sit down to a collage of Gaone cuisines. As the aroma of delectable delights wafted through the house, Steve's older brother Phil yelled, "What staple did Jenna bring?"

Before Jenna could answer Phil, his wife playfully chastised saying, "Obviously not the kind that keeps a rude mouth like yours shut."

Amid the laughter, all eyes shifted to Jenna. In mock seriousness, she surveyed the burgeoning buffet before saying, "I have to admit my shrimp falls short."

Chuckles rippled through the gathering. Phil grabbed Steve's shoulder and said, "I like this one. Try not to screw it up." Patting Steve's cheek, he whispered, "We need to keep Mom quiet."

Steve let out a laugh. "I started sending memos two weeks ago, but short of yanking out her tongue—"

"Tongue removal's useless," Phil countered. "She'd turn life into a constant game of Charades."

Mike congregated with his cousins in front of a popular video game and called out, "Uncle Phil! You want to know what it's like to get," he squeezed his clasped hands together, "crushed?"

Phil puffed out his chest, strutted toward the group of teens, and bragged, "Not a man alive can take me down at this game."

As he positioned himself on a chair readying himself for the match, his younger daughter, Molly, draped her arm on his shoulder and teased, "Didn't Mommy teach you how to play that game last week?"

Amidst some snickering and taunting, he grabbed his daughter in his arms and planted rapid kisses on her face as she tried to wiggle free.

"Be on Daddy's side for a change."

Mike needled, "Come on Uncle Phil; don't listen to that trash talk. Just because ladies and kids can whup yah, that doesn't mean you're all washed up."

Phil eyed Mike and asked, "You wash my car every Saturday for a month if you lose?"

"Do I get to drive your car every Saturday for a month if I win?" Mike countered.

While Phil and Mike negotiated the stakes before the match, Clare motioned Jenna toward the sewing room off the kitchen. Jenna was interested in a quilt Clare was creating by sewing together Mike's athletic t-shirts from the time he was in pee-wee sports to graduation. Jenna picked up the blanket and ran her fingers over the embroidery.

"It must have taken you forever to do this stitching. It's beautiful."

Sipping on warm apple cider, Clare said, "It's cheaper than therapy. Sewing takes my mind off worries." Her eyes surveyed the room. "I lose myself in this place after the world beats up on me all day." Clare took another sip of cider and pointed to her drink. "You should try some of this stuff. It has a woozy quality," she said with a giggle.

As sounds of family fun filtered into the sewing room, Jenna's eye caught a Santa Claus decked out in gambling gear. Pointing to the decoration, she asked, "Does he get to stay on display all year?"

Picking up the gambling Santa perched on the sill, Clare said, "Tony bought him for me on our honeymoon. It was our first trip to Vegas. Now, we make it a yearly pilgrimage."

"Oh my gosh! My parents visit Vegas once a year, too. You guys would have a blast together."

"If I play my cards right tonight, Steve promised to foot the bill for this year's trip."

"How sweet. What's the deal?"

Caught off guard, Clare hesitated long enough for Jenna to stammer, "I'm so . . . I'm out of bounds. What he promised you is none of my business."

She turned to join the other guests when Clare waved her hand and said, "Nonsense, Jenna. It's your business." Looking sheepish, she said, "My kids tell me I have a big mouth. I guess I just proved them right." She blurted out, "I think you're a wonderful girl, and Steve doesn't want me to embarrass him by telling everyone I'm thrilled he's seeing an intelligent, attractive girl from a wonderful family." She gulped her drink and said with resignation, "Now, he can get mad at me; Tony will warn me to stay out of it, and Phil and Susan will shake their heads like I'm hopeless." She slipped into a chair and rubbed her brow. "It's just for years I've prayed . . ." She looked up. "He works hard; he's a good father, and he cares about people. You two are perfect for each other."

Jenna fanned herself with her hand and said, "Wow! I'm flattered."

Before Clare could respond, Tony called, "We're gathering in the Thanksgiving circle."

Clare grabbed Jenna's hand and said with renewed enthusiasm, "It feels so good to be myself again, warts and all. Come on, sweetie; this is my favorite part of the holiday."

Family members and guests jousted for comfortable seating, forcing some late arrivals to carve out areas on the floor where they stretched in ease. The gregarious roomful slowly ebbed to silence, interrupted only by an occasional clearing of throats. Soft, seasonal music became more distinguishable. In a solemn voice, Tony Gaone prayed, "We thank God for allowing family and friends to gather on this day to share love and gratitude for each other."

Proclamations of gratitude continued around the room until all eyes landed on Mike. Lying on the floor, clasping his hands behind his raised head, he said, "I'm thankful I called that parent/teacher conference to convince Miss Rossi that I'm not a cheater." Pointing at her, he said, "Marawski's the one who cheated!"

Amid the laughter, his Uncle Phil teased, "Then explain how you won that lousy computer game with a hundred points more than me, Mikey . . . why I have to fill your tank this week."

Tony pointed to Jenna and said, "Before we cart Phil away to a magical place that teaches him how to lose gracefully, we'd like to hear from you."

Sitting on an ottoman, hugging a pillow to her chest, she smiled at Steve and said, "Ditto Mike." She swung her eyes to Mike, winked, and told him, "I know you're not a cheater." Teasing Phil, she said, "Rumor has it Mike invoked the mercy rule."

Phil complained, "What kind of teacher are you? You just made my self-esteem plummet."

Mike defended Jenna by pointing out, "She's an awesome teacher, Uncle Phil, not a miracle worker."

The raucous made it difficult to hear the phone ringing in Jenna's purse. Clare passed the bag to Jenna and said, "I think it's been ringing off and on for the last five minutes."

Jenna saw that it was Samantha Kind, excused herself, and joyfully sang, "Happy Thanksgiving, Sam."

Mike looked at his father with a Cheshire grin. "We saved the best for last, Dad, but wait for Jenna before you take your turn."

Steve sipped on his wine and shot Jenna a futile look. She waved him to go on without her. He raised his brows and told Mike, "She won't be back for at least fifteen minutes."

The senior Gaone sat back and said, "Tell us what's going on in your head and heart, son."

"This family's given me, given all of us, more than we could ever repay, but what did we ever give the Indians to be thankful for that first Thanksgiving?"

A groan rose from some of the participants giving way to a mass exit in the direction of refreshments beckoning the overstuffed bellies. As some relatives simply shook their heads in dismay, one or two disgruntled aunts and uncles lagged behind to chastise Steve for his over-analysis and ill-timed editorial opinion. Tony pointed at his son and said, "That's why we saved you for last." He pulled himself out of the chair and wrapped Steve in a warm embrace. "An honest answer to that question would ruin Thanksgiving forever."

Nodding, Steve asked, "Where'd Mom disappear to?"

"She's in the kitchen loading the dishwasher," Phil told him. Slapping his brother on the back, he added, "Perfect timing, Stevie. We gave the Indians diseases, and Karma gave us you."

Ignoring his brother's friendly harassment, he intercepted his mother organizing the desserts after the guests tore through the kitchen like a swarm of locusts.

"Jenna and I are heading out." He grabbed her from behind and gave her a soft bear hug. "Get me the dates for Vegas, and I'll book your flight and accommodations."

Without turning around to face his impending wrath, she grabbed the whistling teakettle. "I can't accept your gift, baby."

"Why not?" he asked with indictment.

Drying her hands on her apron, she turned to face him. "Jenna will probably tell you about our talk, so I may as well tell you first."

Frustration mounting, he asked, "What's it going to take for you to stop involving yourself in my love life? Can't you just once let a relationship unfold naturally?" Breaking his cold stare, he asked, "What happened to, 'Have faith things will work out,' you're always preaching?"

Clare was revving up to respond when Jenna, searching for Steve, pushed the kitchen door open and sang out, "There you are." She gave Clare a hug and said, "Thank you for a wonderful evening." The strained look on both their faces told Jenna that she had stumbled into a major disagreement. Before the silence consumed them, she said, "I'm sorry. I'll come back when—"

"No, sweetheart, stay." Clare folded a dish towel and laid it on the counter. "Steve's upset because he believes I'm interfering."

Leaning back on the counter, he crossed his arms over his chest, and shot his mother a stern look. Turning to Jenna, he said, "Let's go." He motioned his head toward the dining room where voices filtered to the kitchen. "Any moment they'll morph into a Gallup Poll on our love-life."

"Do what you want," Clare said, faking nonchalance. "I think it's a compliment that Jenna knows I like her and her family."

Disbelief crossed his face. "I hope I never embarrass Mike the way you embarrass me." He looked at Jenna and asked, "You ready?"

Jenna rested her hand on his forearm and said, "I'd like to add my two cents."

Visibly on edge, he said, "I prefer that you don't."

With a knowing smile, she asked, "Remember what my mother did to us at my family reunion?"

"Indelibly."

She turned to Clare and said, "She dragged your son from one relative to the other and kept repeating, 'He's intelligent, handsome, and highly successful.'" Jenna's sympathetic eyes washed over Steve, curbing his animosity. "At least she listed the euphemism for money last." With mock seriousness, she said, "They could've locked me up in Singsing for the way I tore into her the next day."

Fighting a smile, he placed one hand over his heart and raised the other high over his head. "I swear we're scheduling genetic profiling before we conceive a child. What are the chances the dominant gene responsible for 'foaming at the mouth' isn't hereditary?" Walking toward the back door, he said, "The only way to ensure normality is to adopt."

Placing her hands on her hips, Clare said, "Keep picking on me, and I'll call Rosie right this minute and tell her you're talking babies."

Steve grabbed Jenna's hand. "Let's scram before she calls a priest."

Jenna hugged Clare again. "No matter what he says, he owes you that trip to Vegas."

Steve raised both hands and crossed his index fingers to ward off Clare's attempt to barrage him with good-bye kisses. "No closer, Mom. You did more than enough for me tonight."

Clare grabbed his face and kissed him hard on the cheek. "You ought to know by now that no matter how old you get, Stephen, you and Phil will always be my babies."

At home in her apartment, Jenna nestled in Steve's arms and said, "Even when you're at odds, you and your mother express so much love."

"She pretends to worry about Phil as much as she worries about me, but we both know she can't shake off what happened to me when I was eighteen." He glided his fingers up and down Jenna's arm and admitted, "Sometimes it still scares me." Several moments of silence passed before he said, "She hovers." Taking a deep breath, he exhaled, and said, "The one or two women who caught my interest over the years never fared well with her."

"Does she overstep boundaries?"

Letting out a laugh, he told her, "She's a well-tuned harmony drone capable of zeroing in on blatant incompatibilities. I used to believe people changed for the ones they loved." He rested his head on the back pillow of the couch. "I've learned that people generally stay the same or act worse after growing comfortable in a relationship."

She planted a soft kiss on his cheek and said, "If you ask me, your mom has a sixth sense about the women you encounter."

"Easy for you to say, Rossi. She likes you."

"That's right, Stephen." With an air of superiority, she burrowed deeper into his chest. "And I'll tell yah, cowboy, it feels great to have a mother believe I'm good enough for her precious baby boy."

He pulled back and eyed her. "At what point do you think she should start trusting her baby boy's judgment?"

Shrugging, she said, "You're asking the wrong person. My parents probably believe I'd sleep with any man who tells me I have pretty eyelashes."

"By all means, allow me to attest to your born-again virginity."

Playing with the hair on his arm, she said reflectively, "There's a lot of love behind your mom's badgering." Raising her eyes, she said, "The most touching part of your family's celebration was watching your dad hug you after everyone chorused hisses and boos when you ruined the Thanksgiving circle with that random Indian question."

"You were talking to Sam. I didn't think you noticed."

"I multitask when I listen to her ramble. I've suffered through reruns of her abuse for years, which likely makes me a candidate for second hand PTSD."

"Talk about PTSD," he said laughing, "Ask Phil about how my father scarred him for life because of one simple comment he made at the supper table. My dad grabbed him by his neck and dangled him off the floor for thirty seconds."

"Your mild-mannered father choked Phil?"

Laughing harder, he said, "With one hand! The best part was watching my mother stand in total silence for once in her life."

Pulling her hair to the top of her head and holding it in place with both hands, Jenna asked, "What in God's name did Phil say to rile him?"

"I was ten; he was thirteen. A whiff of my mother's meatloaf from the kitchen would send us finagling an invitation to a friend's house to eat, but that time our luck ran out. Even the maggots in our garbage can felt the same way about her meatloaf as we did. They cleared out for weeks."

"Your mom's an excellent cook."

"No doubt her kitchen's a slice of heaven, but after one bite of her meatloaf, wrestling a two-headed alligator's more appealing than a second bite." Remembering with a smile, he said, "First, Phil gagged, then he blurted out his grand idea to save mankind from all future wars by saying, 'Mom should work for the defense department.' My dad glared at him and ordered him to be quiet, but Phil persisted. 'No, Dad, listen. If the government forced people to eat everything they kill and sprinkled Mom's meatloaf on the dead bodies for seasoning then—' BAM!"

Jenna dropped her hair, stared wide-eyed at Steve, and said, "Oh my gosh! How disgusting."

Palming his chest, Steve laughed hard saying, "In a nanosecond, my father reached across the table, grabbed Phil by the neck, lifted him six inches off the floor, pressed him hard against the wall, and said through clenched teeth, 'If you ever make fun of your mother's cooking again, I'll hurt you.' My dad opened up his hand wide, and Phil dropped to the floor flailing like the Scarecrow on fire in *The Wizard of Oz*."

As Steve fought to catch his breath from laughter, Jenna covered her mouth with her hands and said, "Your mother must've been frantic."

With a loud sigh, Steve said, "She acted like it was standard behavior for my dad to strike out every time we mouthed off. When Phil, dazed by the attack, said, 'Dad tried to kill me! My own father tried to murder me!' my mom wiped some spilled water off the table, straightened the salt and pepper shakers, and said, 'You know better than that, Phillip. If your father wanted to kill you, you'd be dead.'"

Laughing together, Steve pulled Jenna close and played with her hair. "That night we heard my mother and father arguing in their bedroom. My mother yelled, 'You could've hurt him, Tony. Besides, my meatloaf *is* awful. I'm never cooking it again.' My dad told her, 'It's not the meatloaf, Clare. The boys need to learn respect.' There were more heated words before we heard my dad say, 'Thank you for not undermining me in front of them.' Her voice was softer saying, 'I love you, Tony, and the boys love and respect you, too.' Then there was that familiar silence."

"What happened?" she asked full of wonder.

"What always happened, what still happens when they're in their bedroom together for more than three minutes," he said, letting out an incredulous laugh. "They're like college kids in heat. Phil and I used to wonder how we managed to have our own rooms. The way they play around, we could've easily racked up a baker's dozen of siblings." He massaged Jenna's neck and more seriously said, "I never would've made it with Mike after Amy died if my mother wouldn't have forced me to make it." Quiet moments lapsed as Jenna laid her head on his chest and listened to the strong, rhythmic beat of his heart.

Tracing Jenna's face with his fingertip, he told her, "My mother makes waves, but she makes it her mission to help me and Phil keep the water out of the ship." Tilting his head, he asked, "Your parents are loving people. Why didn't you give them a chance to help you with the baby?"

Sitting up, she curled her feet under her, and picked at a pillow. "I know they love me, but when Josh died, I struggled to be like the good, sweet kid they buried. Not only did I fail miserably," her eyes dropped, "I crushed them at their lowest point. They lost Josh, and I gave away their grandchild." Resting her head on her knee, she said, "I don't tell them my problems because I don't want to burden or disappoint them." Her eyes glistening, she said, "I'd give anything for a do-over."

He cuddled her and urged, "Open up a little more. Give them a chance to help you out. Parents live to forgive their kids."

Forcing a smile, she said, "Do you mind if we keep the water outta the ship tonight? Regurgitating my cornucopia of misguided decisions will either make me suicidal or homicidal." She jumped up, turned on the CD player, and broke into a sexy, lascivious dance. Her index finger seductively motioned for him to join her. "Teach me some of your smooth moves, Casanova."

He grabbed hold of her, twirled her around a couple of times, and said, "This is my favorite." Yanking her toward him, he did a little cha-cha, dipped her low, and caused her to tumble softly to the floor dragging him down on top of her. She was laughing uncontrollably when he did a slow push-up off her and said, "Before I teach you the art of dipping, I need to give you something important."

Struggling to suppress her laughter, she took several breaths, tapped his lips, and said, "The only thing these luscious lips need to give me is an apology for ruining the dance."

He pulled back in mock surprise. "You'll have a nursing home address and dentures in a jar before these lips apologize for your inability to dip properly, but—"

"Come on, Stephen! That was the worst dip ever. A simple, 'I'm sorry,' will suffice."

"Stop interrupting, and I'll apologize, not for the bad dip, but for—"

"For what, then? It's not like I'm asking you to apologize for everything you've ever done wrong in your life."

He gently covered her mouth with his hand and said, "I'm sorry that I forgot to give you one of those 'Define What Love Is' essays you assigned the kids to hand in before Thanksgiving vacation." Freeing her mouth, he added, "When you picked up the stack in my car the other day, it must've fallen loose on the back floor." He stood over her, dusted his pants, and said, "I don't want the kid getting downgraded because of me."

She stared up at him in disbelief.

After one hard blink, she said, "While I'm lying at your feet, your romantic reaction to my lusty overture is to hand me an essay?"

Minimizing her belief that he was inattentive to her, he said, "I probably should've waited, but then I was curious about what the kid had to say."

She jumped to her feet and dusted off her pants with hard, deliberate strokes. Unable to hide her hurt feelings, she dealt an uncharacteristic blow.

"Frankly, it might be more appealing to read some kid's tripe than beg a guy for attention." Plopping on the couch, she added, "For someone who graduated in the top ten at Columbia, you—"

"Top five," he corrected her.

His intentional, flippant correction of her inconsequential error unnerved her. She tossed a pillow to the floor and countered, "You irked your family with that ill-timed Indian question; now you're taunting me?"

To avoid an escalation over what Steve perceived as trivial, she said, "We're both tired. Let's call it a night."

Mystified by her over-reaction, he asked, "I didn't feel neglected when you excused yourself from the Thanksgiving circle to listen to Sam, so why the over-sensitivity about a kid's essay interrupting us for five minutes tonight?"

"You expect me to apologize for shining some light into Sam's otherwise bleak world?" Shaking her head, she asked, "Isn't an extended family unloading a heap of thankfulness sufficient to quench your thirst for attention?" She crossed her arms. "At least Sam appreciates me."

"Look," he said more softly. "It might be fun to see what the kid has to say about love. Maybe we can both learn something new."

Refusing to take possession of the paper, she sat back, covered her face with her hands for several seconds, and battled her hurt pride. "I'm sorry, Steve, but reading an essay on Thanksgiving Day isn't on my radar for a romantic evening." Motioning her head toward the table near the door, she said, "Leave it on your way out."

In mild amazement, he tapped the rolled essay on his free, open hand and said, "You're pointing to the door, and I'm pointing to your heart."

His accusatory assessment of her hurt feelings stirred anger in her. She shot back, "I won't feel guilty for refusing to work on Thanksgiving Day."

Intentionally disregarding her heightened perturbation with him, he sat next to her and gently pushed until her head rested on the back of the couch. "Tell you what," he said with misplaced enthusiasm. "I want you to enjoy Thanksgiving. I'll hold you in my arms while you read the essay to me. How's that sound?"

With mounting frustration, she complained saying, "You do this all the time. You did it when you kissed me on the hill; you did it dancing at the Autumn Ball; you did it at—"

"Read to me, Jenna." Pressing his thumb on her lips, he whispered a sultry, "I love when you read to me."

Her eyes pierced him with skepticism. Slowly sitting up, she said, "You win. Give that to me."

"Wait!" He wrapped his arms around her and settled back comfortably. "Now we're ready."

Eyeing him with suspicion, she asked, "Is this some kind of test to see how far you could push me?"

"Only a fool would light the fuse of a powder keg and hold on to it."

A wry smile crossed her lips. "I'm the fool. I should know by now that you're always up to something, Gaone." She flipped open the essay and began to read.

"Juliet speaks in haste when she says of her love, Romeo, 'Take him and cut him out in little stars/And he will make the face of heaven so fine/That all the world will be in love with night/And pay no worship to the garish sun.' The truth is 'the sun' lights and warms the earth like 'love' lights and warms the heart. While the sun may be bold, intense, and garish at times, like love, it is necessary to soothe, sustain, and renew."

After several exaggerated sniffs, she sang, "I smell plagiarism." She flipped the paper back to front in search of the culprit's name.

"Let me help you look."

She shot back saying, "You really want to help? Find an anesthesiologist who's willing to put me under and forget to wake me up."

Winking, he said, "You have miles to go before you sleep."

Nudging him, she asked, "Did you write this?"

He motioned with his hand for her to continue reading.

"Love is like the sun peaking over the horizon. It awakens me to a life full of promise. Love is like the sun at high noon. It commands that I work, play, and burn hot with desire. Love is like the sun setting at twilight. It invites me to tranquil rest."

Her soft eyes falling on him, she said, "This is poetry."

"Really? I thought essays were prose."

Her heart racing, she disregarded his comment and read:

"Even brighter than the sun, love illumines the darkest crevices of my being and lends me courage to hold on one second longer. Love is like the sun that bursts with energy; heat so hot yet indomitably willing to retreat behind soft, billowy clouds when weaker flaws inflame."

Steve felt a slight tremble run through her body as she sat silent for several seconds staring at his declaration of love.

"Don't stop now," he whispered. "The best part's coming up."

"How do you know?"

Taking the essay from her hand, he said, "Because it's what I'd say if I were describing love."

She laid her head on his shoulder and listened to his voice carry her to his heart.

"For these reasons, Juliet is wrong. While all the world falls in love with the stars at night, I love the sun. Unlike distant stars that hang bright and beautiful yet lifeless in the cold, dark sky, my love is like the sun that soothes, sustains, and renews. Jenna is the sun that rises in the East. Jenna is the sun that brightens my world with laughter, learning, and love. Jenna is the sun, and she is necessary."

"I can't stop tingling over every inch of my body."

He held her face and said, "Ahhh! That explains it."

"Explains what?" she whispered.

"I'm tingling, too."

Chapter Ten

EARLY FRIDAY MORNING, JENNA SWUNG BY HER MOTHER'S house to join her aunt and cousin on their traditional Black Friday shopping excursion. Jenna sat at the table and sipped an espresso while her mother loaded butter on a fresh cinnamon bagel for her.

"Not too much, Mom."

"Butter's good for you, Jenna. You're thin."

"My weight's average for my height."

"Tell us about the Gaone Thanksgiving dinner?" her Aunt Jo coaxed as she bit into some fruit.

"Talk about a food-fest," Jenna told them. She looked at her mother and said, "They visit Vegas each year, too." Reaching for a rum cookie, she added, "You guys should plan a trip together."

"Your father and Tony Gaone would have a blast. I enjoy talking to Clare when I have the chance. They're nice people."

Licking her fingers, Jenna said, "They feel the same about our family."

Rosie handed Jenna a napkin. "I hope you used one of these when you were sitting at their table."

Licking her thumb with exaggerated force, she said, "Whatever I did there must have worked, because Steve's mother loves me."

"That guy's so gorgeous," her cousin Gabby chimed in. "He's worth a girl forgetting her birth control pills."

Jenna locked eyes with her mother. Stunned by the closeness of the taboo topic, Rosie turned to use her work at the sink to camouflage her shock.

"What kind of ass-backward attitude to build a loving relationship is that?" Jenna's Aunt Jo yelled at her daughter. "How can any of you girls find a decent man when it doesn't bother you that dogs show more respect for their females than some men do? It doesn't help when women run around showing cleavage down to their vaginas, either!"

"Sounds like someone forgot to take a different kind of pill this morning," Gabby said, needling her mother. "Like I'm really going to rush out and get pregnant to hook a guy." Biting into her bagel, she added, "Still, if I had cleavage, I'd be showing it, and if I were Jenna, I'd send Steve a thank you note for making every woman she knows jealous."

Rosie dried her hands with a dish towel, turned to her niece, and said, "We're going to have fun shopping like we do every year, Gabrielle. Your mother and I may not agree with all the new-fangled lifestyles of the younger generation, but don't you ever forget that we'd love and support you even if you did something as half-assed backward as get pregnant before you get married."

Gabby jumped up, wrapped her arms around her aunt, and declared, "I love you, Aunt Rosie; I love this whole crazy family."

Jenna smiled at her mother and mouthed, "Thank you."

Starlight beamed off the blue Forrester as Jenna's aunt and cousin loaded up the car with a small mountain of Christmas treasures. After the lingering goodbye hugs and kisses, Gabby nudged her mother toward the car. "Stop acting like you're being separated by the Berlin Wall for fifty years. Tomorrow you'll be together baking cookies from eight in the morning 'til eight at night."

Rosie grabbed Gabby's face, kissed it hard, and said, "I used to think they called you Gabby because it was cute."

"Love you, Aunt Rosie." She waved goodbye to Jenna and said, "Call me."

Jenna sat at the kitchen table with her mother and shared a cup of tea. With a hint of worry, Rosie asked, "Do you want to talk about it?"

Playing with her spoon, Jenna said, "I want to share something with you, Mom."

Rosie cupped her warm mug and said, "I'm listening, baby."

Jenna pulled Steve's essay from her purse and slid it across the table. "What do you think of this?"

Rosie reached for her glasses and scanned the first paragraph. Raising her eyes over the rims, she cautioned, "If a student wrote this, you better nip it in the bud."

Jenna motioned for her to keep reading.

Rosie raised her hand to her mouth to stifle a soft gasp. "He loves you!" Looking up, she asked, "Does he know?"

Jenna assured her. "I told him everything weeks ago, Mom." Palming the essay, she said, "He knows who I am, and he loves me."

Claiming relief, Rosie held Jenna's face and kissed her on both cheeks. "He's a lucky man, baby, and don't you forget it." More subdued, she said, "Please go slow. It won't hurt to learn more about each other."

"Steve has reasons to be just as careful as I do." Sipping her tea, she said, "It's no secret he married his wife because she was pregnant. This time, he's in it for love."

Dominic Rossi waded through the boxes and bags on his way to the kitchen. "Do I have to get a second job to pay for all that merchandise in the foyer?"

Rosie grabbed him by his belt buckle and planted a soft kiss on his cheek. "A couple of those gifts are for you, big guy." Turning to Jenna, she said, "Tell your father the good news."

His eyes held Jenna as he wrapped his arms around his wife and squeezed. "What's new, princess?"

Gazing at her parents with admiration, she said, "I hope Steve, someday, loves me as much as you love Mom."

Rosie waved Steve's letter and said, "He's off to a good start."

Dom asked, "What's that?"

"Steve told me he loves me."

Dom waved Jenna into his arms and rocked her and Rosie back and forth. He whispered in measured tone, "That man has good taste." Kissing Jenna's forehead, he reminded her, "I loved you first."

Despite his playful posturing, Jenna was keenly aware of her father's unspoken reservations. She eyed him with child-like desire to be accepted and said, "I want you both to know that neither of us wants a repeat of our past mistakes."

Concern gradually slipped from their faces. Dom pecked her on the cheek and retreated to the den while Jenna and her mother talked a while longer. Glancing at the clock, Jenna grabbed her purse and fumbled for her keys.

"I better head home and get some rest. Steve wants to check out that gigantic mall they built in Lexington. I'd like to carve out some time to spend with Sam this weekend, too."

"How's that poor soul these days? Every time I think of that Brad Kind . . ." Rosie shook her head in disgust.

"She's the same. All she does is cry and mull over why her parents hurt her."

Rinsing the mugs, Rosie said, "Memories hold us hostage. Some days, the good ones are no match for the bad." She turned around and said, "I'll never forgive myself for not following up with Child Protective Services after they moved away."

Jenna's brows rose. "You did everything you could, Mom. You practically let Sam live with us until they forbade her from visiting." Jenna let out a laugh. "Remember how no matter what kind of pasta we were eating on Sundays, you'd cook Sam a small bowl of angel hair pasta and tell her she was our visiting angel? Even after her mother ended the visits, Josh would sneak the pasta to her. To this day she tells me you're the only one who ever made her feel special."

Turning to dry the mugs, Rosie said, "I'll never forget that day she was in your bedroom trying on the clothes you outgrew. I popped in to see how you girls were doing. When I gave her a big hug, I noticed bruises. I just about fainted." Rosie twisted the towel tightly in her hands and said, "Someone should've strangled that beast! Animals live better than they allowed that beautiful girl to live."

"I was the last to know what was happening with her," Jenna mused. "Sam told me the bruises were from hiking and falling off her bike. I believed her, because what did I know?" Making her way back to the table, she added, "Now she tells me the stories over and over again. It's like her father abused both of us."

"I suspected Brad, but I never in a million years thought Brenda would turn a blind eye. They both had to be insane. What kind of people cause their child to witness death?" She sat across from Jenna and said, "I should have contacted Child Protective Services the first time I saw those bruises. A week after I finally contacted them, the family picked up and moved away. Just like that!" Rosie said, snapping her fingers. "God help me, Jen, I should've followed up. It was around the time we lost Josh, and I was wrapped up in my own pain."

Jenna hugged her mother and said, "If everyone had a heart as wide as yours, there'd be less pain in the world. You and Dad are always open to people in need. Trust me; by the time Sam was out of grade school, her parents turned her heart into a sieve."

Walking to the door together, Rosie said, "Never underestimate the healing power of reaching out to someone, baby. Our simple acts of kindness are God's answers to people's prayers."

Jenna turned to her mother and said, "If I were Sam, I would've killed them both long before she pulled that trigger."

"It's hard not to feel that way, because all that girl needed was a hug now and then, some positive attention to give her some self-worth."

"Well, I need a hug good-bye," Jenna said, planting a kiss on her mother's cheek and calling out good-bye to her father. "Talk to you tomorrow."

Rosie turned off the bedroom lamp and rolled into Dominic's arms. "She's finally going to be okay."

Dominic countered in a faint voice, "How can any of us ever be okay when a part of us is somewhere out there?"

"Jenna's reconciled with her choice, Dom. We have to have faith that the child's thriving." Rosie's eyes watered. "Jenna knows how hurt we are; she knows we would've fought to raise the baby. We can't keep allowing one horrible decision to cloud all the positives she accomplishes." Fluffing her pillow, she told him, "We need to stop our sadness from casting shadows on her life."

He pulled her close. "I've learned to live with knowing I can't resurrect Josh, but knowing that baby's out there and I'm not a part of her life cuts like a knife through my heart."

Morning came quickly, and after hours of battling crowds curious to inspect the new mega mall in the area, Jenna flung her apartment door open and allowed Steve, balancing several boxes of Christmas gifts, to walk through first. She quickly followed and piled her bags near the couch, slipped out of her boots, and dropped with fatigue. Looking up at him, she said, "You're almost as much fun on a shopping spree as the Rossi ladies."

"Whoever said nothing lasts forever didn't take into account the glut of commercialism that disguises as Christmas shopping."

"Christmas is never long enough, Steve."

"Are you kidding? The shopping season begins the day after Halloween and ends at Easter."

"I take it back," she said with a laugh. "You're not as fun as my mom and aunt."

Pressing his knee into the couch cushion, he gently tumbled on top of her, and teased, "Yeah, but I offer better post-shopping amenities."

His lips surfed her face, planting soft kisses on her cheeks, neck, and lips. His hand slipped under her shirt and massaged her chest for several seconds before sliding back to loosen her bra. He glided back to her chest and gently fumbled one of her breasts. A soft groan rose from her before she gave him a gentle shove and said, "Don't get carried away, cowboy. I'll have to throw you in a cold shower."

His body hovering inches above her, he whispered in a low excited voice, "I'll know when to stop, Jen. Trust me. We can shower afterwards."

"I do trust you, Steve." With a more forceful push, she sat up, took a deep breath, and pulled her hair back. "We have to do it right this time. We both know what an unplanned pregnancy can do to a relationship."

He rolled to a sitting position and rested his head on the back pillow. Still breathing heavily, his voice filled with anticipation. "We bought a lot of gifts tonight, but the only thing I want is you."

"I'm not a *thing*," she reminded him. With a soft stare, she added, "Ever since I gave my baby up, I associated those words from every overly eager man I dated with impending doom." Running her fingertips over the back of his hand, she told him, "You've become the center of my world. Gravity keeps pulling me into your arms." She gently kissed his lips and said, "Not only do I trust you; I love you. I feel safe with you. That's why I'm still with you."

"Why do I detect the word *but* floating around on that luscious tongue of yours waiting to tumble out and break my heart?"

She tenderly surveyed his face before saying, "Your essay impressed my parents."

"But?"

"But they still can't forget what happened the last time I believed a guy loved me."

Stiffening his jaw, he muttered, "I'm nothing like Ronan King."

"You wouldn't be sitting on my couch if I didn't recognize the distinct difference between you and Ronan King."

Eyeing him more thoughtfully, she said, "I told them how I feel about intimacy, and within reason, I want to see it through."

"Let me guess, Jen. The chastity belt doesn't come off until you have a ring on your finger and a ring through my nose?"

Taking umbrage with his acerbic attitude toward marriage, she countered, "If you view commitment to me as a life of confinement and servitude, revise that essay for someone more compatible."

More hurt than angry, she stood to walk away, but Steve grabbed her leg causing her to buckle and fall back onto the couch. He told her, "It's a cinch to revise the essay, but even a transplant wouldn't be able to revise my heart." Resting his head on the back pillow, he asked in a more conciliatory tone, "So, what should I expect moving forward?"

For a moment, she thought of holding back, but love and respect for him made truth easy. "I want to make sure that the next child I bring into the world has the unconditional love of a mother and father who conceived it."

He clasped his hands behind his head and dared her to find fault with his logic. "I share your sentiment, so let's explore ways to share intimacy and prevent pregnancy until we're ready for parenthood."

Rolling her eyes, she asked, "Aren't you forgetting a step?"

Steve leaned back and quickly assessed their relationship. He fought a smile that tried to creep onto his face. Pointing his finger at her, he said, "First you tie me up with these archaic regulations about sex. Now, you're finagling a marriage proposal. Do you have a problem with my reserving the right to hold on to some small piece of my manhood?"

She straddled him and said seductively, "Poor baby. I didn't mean to strip you of your," her eyes fell to his groin, "manhood. If I would've known you stored the essence of your being in that little male organ—"

"Careful what you're calling little, Jen. The only people who claim size doesn't matter are the ones who lack endowment." Reaching for his zipper, he said, "I have no qualms about providing you proof of your erroneous assessment of my—"

Grabbing his hand, she laughed, and said, "I'm sure the Penis Museum in Iceland has nothing over you, but let's spend quality time exploring reasonable ways to share intimacy without procreating. That should restore the manhood I callously robbed from you."

Caught off guard by her willingness to abandon her previous abstinence pledge, Steve nodded approvingly.

Jenna added, "If you're as good as you claim, and we someday . . ." Catching herself in mid-sentence, she said, "We can vacation in Iceland and visit some of your heroes."

Surveying her body with hungry eyes, he pulled her toward him and gently assaulted her face with soft kisses. He swept her mouth with his tongue. Moving back up to her neck, he planted several more kisses below her ear and whispered, "I've negotiated hundreds of deals but none as pleasurable as this one."

She grabbed his face with both hands and kissed him hard on the lips. Gently tracing the lines on his face with her index finger, her eyes sized him up before she said, "I never thought a man would love me enough to meet my unconventional demands so easily."

Wrapping his arms around her, he said, "I never thought a woman existed who made waiting this long worth my while." Tilting his head, he asked, "Is there really a penis museum in Iceland?"

Letting out a sensuous laugh, she said, "There sure is, cowboy."

With bravado, he told her, "Someday I'll be in that museum."

"Only if I buy you a ticket," she teased.

"I've been trying to show you my ticket for months."

Chapter Eleven

SPORTSMEN'S *GUN AND GAME EXTRAVAGANZA*, ONE OF THE SCHOOL'S annual events, displayed myriad weapons, taxidermy techniques, and conservation seminars, a large draw for outdoor enthusiasts in the tri-state area. There were games, prizes, concessions, and notable speakers with expertise in the fields of hunting, conservation, and game food preparation. Jenna was one of the coordinators for the ticket sales and concession stands. She was elated when Steve volunteered to help.

Standing at the bottom of his steps, Steve hollered up to his son, "The clock's ticking, Mike."

Bounding down the stairs, he said, "Geez, Dad! You wouldn't move this fast if you were a driver in the Indy 500. No woman's ever doing that to me."

Before Steve turned to open the door, he said, "For the record, Michael, I didn't let just any woman transform me from a Neanderthal to the epitome of the male species that I am." Patting Mike's cheek, he said, "I'll remind you of this conversation when your heart's hooked on some worthwhile beauty. Until then, keep moving before Jenna dumps me for a guy who knows how to tell time."

When they arrived at the school, young and old waded in and out of rooms that appealed to their personal interests. Wild turkeys gobbling and dogs barking drew the attention of hundreds of hunting enthusiasts.

"Ty's driving tonight, Dad. I have my key."

"You know the drill, Mike. My phone's on."

Mike nodded then disappeared into the moving mass of humanity.

"Steve!" Jenna called, waving from across the gymnasium. "I need you to collect entry fees at the main gate."

"I'm your man," he said, grinning.

"I like the sound of that," she said, patting him on the chest. Before he could grab hold of her, she floated away saying, "Mr. Foster will explain the procedure. I need to check the concession stand." Blowing him a kiss, she vanished as quickly as she appeared.

As soon as an irate parent spotted Jenna, she pointed to several unruly students who grabbed three bottles of water but refused to pay. Jenna turned to see Stewart Jones sitting under the stairwell with two of his younger friends drinking the stolen water. As she walked toward them, they whispered and laughed.

"Hey guys, you owe Mrs. Dean for that water. Make it right, okay?"

Stewart's lewd stare unnerved her. Without blinking, he said, "I'll pay for the water if you answer a question."

"I don't have time for games, Stew."

"Does Mr. Gaone pay for what he gets, or do you give it to him for free?"

Jenna's face flushed.

Registering shock at Stewart's implication, his friends turned to him and warned, "Shut up, man! She'll kick us out!"

Stewart held Jenna in his defiant stare. She swung her controlled anger to the underclassmen and said, "Pay for your water and don't cause any more trouble. Expect a detention slip Monday morning." Turning to Stewart, she said, "I've always treated you with respect, but respect works both ways. I'll give you a chance to walk that comment back before I hold you accountable for sexual harassment."

Stewart stared unflinchingly, swallowed more water, and laughed.

Jenna scanned the crowd and caught Marcus Wright talking to a parent sitting at a table in the concession area. She waved him to the stairwell.

"What's the problem here?" he asked, eyeing Stewart Jones sitting on a wooden crate nonchalantly screwing the cap onto the water bottle.

Struggling to keep an even tone, Jenna's eyes blazed.

"Stew refuses to pay for that water he picked up at the concession stand. I asked him and his two friends to make it right, but instead, Stew chose to harass me with sexual innuendo."

Marcus swung his eyes to Stewart. "I'd like to hear your side of it, Stew."

With a pasted smirk on his face, he asked, "Can't you take a joke?"

Marcus swung his eyes to Jenna. "Can you take a joke, Miss Rossi? Because if you can't take Stewart's joke, he's going to have a major problem on his hands."

Hands on her hips, she told Stewart, "Sexual harassment and defamation of character aren't jokes."

Marcus eyed the fidgeting student. "She's right, Stew. A bad joke gets you three days; sexual harassment may get you expelled. What exactly did you say and do?"

With a fixed glare, Jenna answered for him. "He insinuated that Mr. Gaone and I trade sex for money."

Marcus's face paled. "Let's finish this conversation in my office. I'll contact Mr. Jones."

Before Marcus turned to follow Stewart to the office, Jenna said, "The other boys stood down. I'll issue them slips on Monday. I tried to get Stew to back off from that comment, but he was belligerent and adamant." Worried, she told Marcus, "I don't know how Steve will react to Stewart's comment."

Marcus assured her, "He knows how to handle himself. Take a deep breath and come back with him." Before he walked away, he added, "You can't reach them all, Jen. Steve and Mike need to know what happened. Chances are the other boys already texted the whole city."

Jenna explained the circumstances to her co-chairperson and asked that she assume her duties. Walking briskly through the crowded corridors, she entered the front lobby where Steve was amiably collecting the fees. She grabbed another volunteer to replace him and asked Steve to follow her to Marcus's office.

"The principal's office? I wasn't here long enough to do anything wrong," he joked.

As they walked to the principal's office, she said, "We need to find Mike. I want him with us."

Worry crossed Steve's face. He grabbed Jenna's elbow and asked, "What's this have to do with Mike?"

Standing outside the office, Jenna said, "Promise me you'll stay calm. Things like this happen with kids all the time. Marcus will straighten it out."

"Is Mike in trouble?"

"No. I just want Mike and you to hear what happened from me, not from social media."

Just as she began to explain, Mike called to his father. "Dad, I'm glad I found you." His face piqued; his voice shaking, he said, "Everyone's talking about how Stewart Jones is getting suspended for saying you pay Miss Rossi for . . ." He stopped and swung his eyes to Jenna.

"I pay her for what?"

Steve no sooner asked the question when his face flushed. Before he could react to the accusation, Marcus opened his office door and said, "Stewart's father is on his way. I have Stew in here; you guys sit tight out there."

Steve eyed Jenna apologetically. "You warned me about something like this happening." Turning to Mike, he asked, "Are you okay?"

Calmed by his father's low-keyed reaction to the altercation, Mike nodded. Offering consolation, he told Jenna, "All the kids know what he said, but they think Stewart's an idiot. We all respect you." He told his father, "They know you love each other, Dad."

Steve said, "That's a fact." Draping his arm over Mike's shoulders, he asked, "Are you going to be able to handle the goofballs who tease you? It's good to battle for someone's honor, but this . . ." His voice trailed off.

"They've said things before."

Wide-eyed, Steve asked, "When were you going to tell me about it?"

"Geez, Dad! If I told you every rotten thing someone said and did to me, you'd home-school me for the rest of my life."

A half-smile claimed Steve's face. "More likely a private school."

"Private schools have their share of loud-mouth idiots, too, Dad."

Calmed by the absence of anger in his father, he said, "I can handle teasing, but I don't want to handle you going to jail because you punched Stewart's brainless head."

Jenna said, "I have to admit, I was worried about your reaction, too."

"I'm smoldering, but I know physical force won't change the dynamics of this situation for the better. We'll let Marcus handle it."

Jenna touched Mike's shoulder. "It may diffuse the rumors if you're with your friends."

Steve agreed saying, "Call if you need me."

Squeals of excitement from children playing games in the cafeteria and music from the auditorium filtered into the principal's waiting room as Mike opened the door to join his friends talking to a group of girls passing out prizes to the children with winning tickets.

About five-eleven and sporting a beer-belly, a disheveled Mr. Jones burst through the door like an angry bull trapping himself in an undersized room. Prepared to indulge his disdain for any form of authority, he bellowed, "Where's my son?"

Marcus jumped up and said, "I expect civility and respect, Mr. Jones. The inability to exercise both is why we're here in the first place."

"Where's the respect for my son? What the hell did he say that wasn't true?"

Rather than lunge at the loud-mouthed bully standing before him and extracting his vocal chords with his bare hands, Steve pulled back, eyed Mr. Jones, and with premeditated calm said, "One glaring falsehood is your son's claim that I pay Miss Rossi for sex." Verbalizing the insidious accusation left a vile taste in his mouth.

Undaunted by Steve's aggressive defense, Mr. Jones continued to badger. "Guys like you throw money around to get what you want." Scowling, he asked, "Why else would she be so accommodating?"

Steve glanced at Jenna, then swung back to Mr. Jones. Cutting words easily rolled off his tongue. "Maybe she has good taste."

Caught off guard by Steve's derisive response, Mr. Jones turned to Marcus Wright and yelled, "Now ain't that a wholesome way to talk in front of my kid. I suppose he deserves a medal for being civil."

Marcus slammed his hand on the desk. "Be realistic, Mr. Jones. Stewart accused an upstanding teacher of prostituting herself, and her friend, who has an impeccable reputation, defended his and her honor without raising his voice. You, on the other hand, barged in here bolstering your son's false, and I might add, slanderous claim. Don't you see something wrong with this picture?"

"What I see are big shots planning to pin their problems on my kid. Well, expect a fight every step of the way." Mr. Jones glared at his son and motioned his head toward the door. Yanking the door open, he snapped, "Let's get outta here!"

The frolicking sounds of the festivities contrasted with the hostile stand-off taking place in the office. Marcus jumped up, slammed the door shut, and blocked the Joneses from leaving.

"Make no mistake," he warned. "One way or the other, Stewart's outta here." Pointing to Jenna, he said, "Our best bet is to persuade this teacher to be lenient." He looked at Mr. Jones and said, "A ten-day suspension will send the message that students can't slander people without consequences, and we bring Stew back with enough time to make up work and graduate. Walk out that door, you'll be inviting a hearing with the Board of Education." Marcus tossed his pen on the desk. "The Board holds a zero-tolerance policy for sexual harassment. Stew will likely face expulsion for the remainder of the school year." Sitting on the edge of his desk, Marcus pleaded, "For God's sake, let us help your son learn a lesson. If he pulls this garbage out there," he pointed to the street, "they'll fire him or throw him in jail."

Rather than express gratitude for the leniency the principal was offering his son, Mr. Jones ignited with more anger.

"You can't stop my kid from graduating!" he shouted.

Marcus pointed at Mr. Jones and said, "Stewart was out of line, and your defense of his insolent behavior is even more out of line."

Jenna examined the disturbed young man sitting across from her and said, "Tell me what I did or said that causes you to dislike me so much. I'd like to apologize if I hurt you in any way."

Working hard to deflect her kindness, Stewart jumped up saying, "I'm outta here!"

Mr. Jones followed on his heels.

Visibly shaken, Jenna asked, "Am I over-reacting, or is that young man's behavior scary?"

Marcus said, "He's raging. Frankly, I'm surprised he didn't lash out sooner." Tapping his pen on the desk, he asked, "Do you want to give him ten days, or do you want the Board to rule?"

"Let's go with ten days. Stew can't afford to miss more school." Jenna's eyes fell on Steve. "There's a deep-seated hatred for me, and I don't even know why?"

"He's jealous," Steve told her.

"Of what?"

"He's a kid who wants to be proud of his father, but he's smart enough to know that his dad will never attract a woman of your caliber. He's angry with you for choosing to be with Mike's father instead of his father. The father said as much."

Steve walked toward the window and followed the passersby as they moved in and out of the building. More reflective, he said, "My smart-ass comment probably stoked the flames."

Marcus ran his hand through his hair and said, "Make Mike aware of how Stewart feels. Tell him to keep it to himself, but expect the unexpected from that kid. The Jones family's riddled with emotional problems. The mother took off around a year ago, and last Christmas, Stewart's father hauled him in front of the District Justice for knocking out his tooth on Christmas Day. Stew's defense? He said he was tired of his father getting smashed and smacking him around."

"Do you think Stewart will try to hurt Mike?" Jenna asked with worry.

Massaging his forehead with his fingertips, Marcus said, "When we're dealing with unreasonable, angry people, it pays to be proactive." He stood, walked to the door, and said, "We'll keep a close eye on Stew when he comes back from suspension."

Before switching off the lights, he stopped short, breathed in the smell of carnival food, and listened to the laughter. His intuition told him that the gala would end successfully, but the stand-off with the Jones family had only just begun.

Chapter Twelve

"SPRING HAS SPRUNG," FLASHED ON THE MARQUEE IN FRONT of the school. Accompanying the warm, April weather was a serious case of spring fever which complicated Jenna's revision assignment. As she methodically distributed the graded research papers, she worried that the intoxicating sunshine would deter her students from working to their potential.

"If you want to earn one-fourth the amount of points you lost," she told them, "submit your revisions no later than next Monday." She palmed Stewart Jones's empty desk. "Does anyone know if Stew is ill?"

Ahmad was quick to say, "I talked to him last night at the baseball game. He looked okay to me. He said he was doing something with his old man today." Ahmad shot Ken Miller an eye-roll. "Some guys have all the luck."

Careful not to verbalize her disagreement with Ahmad, she thought, I'd hardly call a kid with an abusive father lucky. Instead, she told the class, "If you talk to Stew and any other classmates who are absent today, let them know I'll be at school this Thursday evening from six to eight to help with revisions. Don't wait until the last minute."

As she completed her final instructions at the sound of the bell, Ahmad approached Jenna's desk and asked, "How can a kid come to school every third day and still graduate, Miss Rossi?"

She shuffled some papers into a pile and bound them together with a large paper clip before saying, "Students who miss excessively usually don't graduate."

"You mean Stew's not graduating with us?"

"I didn't say that, and I won't discuss another student's status with you. Get to your next class before the bell rings."

The day passed uneventfully until Mike intercepted Jenna as she was walking to her car at the end of the day.

"Is it true?"

"Is what true?" she asked, slipping her briefcase on the back seat of her car.

"That Stewart's not graduating with us."

"You guys still have two months to go. It's like a football game. A lot can happen before the clock runs out, so I'd advise you to tell everyone to keep working."

"Ahmad told us you said Stewart wasn't graduating because a person can't miss that much school and still graduate."

Rolling her eyes, she said, "Ahmad doesn't listen. I told him it's unusual for someone to miss a lot of school and still graduate, but we always work with kids to get them through." She pushed her hair back and asked with aggravation in her voice, "Where's Ahmad now? He needs to stop talking about Stew before he riles Mr. Jones."

"Ahmad's home, but some of the guys already texted Stew. He said if he's not graduating, there's no sense in wasting his time coming to school."

She held her head and let out a loud, "Grrr!"

Surveying the grassy field ahead of her, she grappled with the distaste of phoning Mr. Jones to explain the misunderstanding. Dragging, her weary body back into the school, she tapped on Marcus's closed door.

"Enter at your own risk."

When she pushed open the door, he quipped, "What took you so long? I heard the rumor an hour ago."

"I never said Stewart wasn't graduating. Ahmad asked a general question about attendance. He applied my general answer to a specific student." Girding herself for a likely battle with Mr. Jones, she asked, "How do I explain an innocent misunderstanding to *Angry Man of the Year*?"

"You don't." He stood and grabbed his jacket. "Right now, I have an appointment with the dentist. I'll call Mr. Jones from home tonight.

I'll already have a headache, so I might not notice the added pounding in my brain." Switching off the lights, he said, "I'll deal with Ahmad first thing tomorrow morning."

After a hellish week of several unpleasant conversations with Mr. Jones, who made every effort to convince anyone who would listen that Jenna didn't plan to help Stewart graduate, she finally convinced him to send his son to school. With Steve on a business trip until late Sunday night, Jenna savored the weekend, carving out time to indulge in a lone shopping spree that provided much needed respite from the barrage she faced all week. Bliss ended when Samantha Kind, oblivious to Jenna's need to ready herself for work, woke her Monday morning ten minutes before the alarm sounded.

Jenna reminded Sam repeatedly, "I can't talk in the mornings when I have school."

Disregarding Jenna's concern, her high-pitched voice cried, "Ikeep" her voice stuck in her throat, "tryin' so hard ta forget. Know why I hate watchin' *I Dream of Jeannie* reruns on television? My mother use ta turn it up reeeally loud. She didn't want to hear me cry when my father . . . She knew he was hurtin' me," she sobbed. "All the while I could hear her laughin' at that fuckin' genie." In between child-like sniffles, she said, "I use ta wish and wish and wish so hard I could find a genie in a bottle. I would've wished them away, wished myself away." Pleading like a child, she cried, "Why me?" She blew her nose hard and said, "My analyst's helping me remember. Ohhh yeah. It's all resurfacing. They ruined my life, Jen. I'll never get a chance to . . . Who cares anyway? Sex is overrated. Everyone screws everyone. Parents screw kids; neighbors screw neighbors' kids, and the government . . . The government fucks us all. I coulda been a proctologist. Been 'round assholes all my life. They made me their huge asshole all my life." After a few more whimpers, she mumbled, "Whocaresanyway?"

Jenna brushed her teeth as she listened to Sam on speaker phone. Rinsing her mouth, she garbled through bubbles and suds, "Icare 'bout you." Swishing her mouth with cold water, she added, "There's plenty of time ta get married and have kids."

Sam said, "My analyst's trying . . . She's trying really hard to help me remember," a burp escaped her, "what they did to me."

"You know how I feel about that lady," Jenna countered, as she lined her eyes and brushed her lashes with mascara. "It's bad enough you agonize over what you actually remember. Why torture yourself over events that may never have happened?"

"Are you saying I should stop seeing her?" Sam asked with hope in her voice.

"Not at all. It's important for you to talk to a professional, but just don't be too quick to let that analyst you're seeing right now talk you into believing something happened that may not have happened. I wish you'd let me help you find a reputable psychiatrist."

Glancing at the clock, Jenna said, "Oh gosh! I'm late; I need to run, Sam."

"Puhleeze, Jen. Talk to me. Sometimes I think everyone will be better off if I just die."

Out of time to play counselor and be sympathetic to the repetitious gory details, she said, "Not now, Sam. Don't start your threats. I'll need to notify the police if you talk suicide. Besides, if you weren't here, I'd lose my hero. I really need to go."

"Hero, hell! Besides, you don't need to go; you choose to go!" she yelled.

Frustration mounted, causing Jenna to yell back, "You're right, Samantha. I choose to be a good teacher. I'm sorry you lost your job, but I still have mine, and I plan to work to the best of my ability. I'll call you tonight and we can—"

Before Jenna could finish her thought and hang up, Sam beat her to it.

Jenna wiggled into her black body briefer, pulled a red, lightweight sweater over her head, and slipped into a pair of black knit pants. She ran downstairs and caught herself in the hallway mirror. Good gosh, she thought. On a scale of professional to sultry, I look like a slut.

"I don't have time for this," she mumbled, scrambling up the stairs, ripping off her sweater and pants and flinging them on the bed. She slipped into a straight, black and white, polka dot dress and jumped into bright, red heels. Snatching a long black and white beaded necklace with three bright red beads to make the outfit pop, Jenna hurried down the stairs, grabbed her purse and keys, and bolted out the door.

Chapter Thirteen

JENNA'S MONDAY MORNING WAS ROUTINE EXCEPT FOR BEGINNING each class period by collecting the revised research papers she assigned the week before. One by one, she dismissed excuses from students who failed for one reason or another to follow directions or submit revisions at all.

One student with uncombed hair and bloodshot eyes said, between a wide yawn, "Last night, we were in the emergency room with my grandfather."

"I'm sorry about your grandfather, John, but you had all week to revise. I urged all of you to avoid conflicts by not waiting until the last minute to complete your work."

He shrugged.

Katie mustered indignation, laying blame on the local college. "They close the library doors at six on Sunday, Miss Rossi. I only had time to find two bibliographies for my paper. Is that okay?"

"What if last week you asked me to write you a letter of recommendation to help you get into Penn State University and I waited until last night to write the letter? I left out several vital facts about you because I carelessly forgot your curriculum vitae at school. You needed the recommendation today, so I just gave you what I had. Is that okay?" Addressing the class, she asked, "Why are you making excuses for mediocrity when you had plenty of time to do your best?" Shaking her head, she told them, "I won't apologize for expecting you to follow directions and put forth your best effort." She exaggerated, "Okay?"

Shyla, a bright and compliant student who had a knack for telling people what they wanted to hear, said, "I don't like all the silly rules and regulations you place on our assignments, like our name, period, and date, have to be in the top right corner of every paper, but my cousin, a college freshman, even said some professors are sticklers that way." Shrugging, she pandered saying, "I guess you're preparing us for college, so, thanks for being bossy, Miss Rossi."

Jenna laughed at her long-winded, back-handed compliment. As she placed the last research paper in a box in front of the room, she turned to the class and teased, "You guys are fortunate that I'm a benign dictator. Now let's get busy learning in Rossi Land."

Her eyes quickly canvassed the class and paused on Stewart Jones who was sitting up straighter than he ever had before. An awkward movement of his hand toward the inside of his shirt made Jenna uneasy. She instinctively moved toward him. His cold, calculated voice ordered, "Take one more step and I'll blow your head off!" The black Glock 23 pistol he pointed at her face was convincing when he said, "It's time we take back our class from the bitchy benign dictator."

There was a ripple of nervous laughter from the students. Ken Miller, sitting in the front seat next to the wall, said, "Come on, Stew. Put that thing away. If you hurt anyone, they'll kick you out for good."

"This isn't the football field, Kenny. You're not calling the shots. I am. Shut your mouth, or I'll shove this in your hole and blow the top of your head off!"

Several girls sniffled louder as Jenna glimpsed Ahmad in the back row looking down, as though he were shooting off a text. After several reprimands for failing to keep his phone in the locker, this time she was grateful for Ahmad's disregard.

Miranda Haney, lounging in her study hall, gasped when Ahmad's text alerted her. "Stew has a gun—hostages."

Texting back at lightning speed, she asked, "joking?"

Ahmad shot back with equal speed, "no!"

Miranda darted across the room to Mrs. Keating's desk. "I don't want to get in trouble for texting, but Ahmad just said Stewart Jones has a gun in Miss Rossi's room."

With subdued caution, the teacher asked to see the messages. Miranda handed the phone to Mrs. Keating and watched the teacher's face pale. Mrs. Keating grabbed her phone and alerted the principal.

Marcus Wright palmed his head. "Are you sure Stewart Jones is involved?"

"The text is clear."

"We're going to lockdown. I'll notify the police."

He checked the class list and circled Mike Gaone's name. After he followed all emergency protocols, Marcus phoned Stephen Gaone.

"Stewart Jones is holding Jenna's classroom hostage. I can't confirm any other details." To alleviate some of Steve's anxiety, Marcus added, "Jenna's smart and gutsy. She knows how to handle these kids."

Steve's world stopped turning.

Unsure of when the first responders would arrive and move into action, Jenna forced eye contact and conversation with Stewart to deflect his attention from the students who were savvy enough to text helpful information to the outside world. Working to keep her voice even and kind, she said, "I know you're angry, Stew, but we can talk this out. You like all these kids. Let them go. Make this between you and me, okay?"

Stewart walked up close to her and snarled like a mad dog poked and teased one too many times. "It's not okay, bitch. From now on, I'll tell you what's okay and what's not okay, OKAY?" he yelled, pressing his face into her face.

The smell of whiskey dizzied her.

He ordered the students with the wave of his gun. "Everyone stand up and move real slow into that corner."

Jenna pointed to the class and yelled, "No! Stay in your seats!"

She knew if Stewart herded the bodies into one large group, not only would he have the capacity to shoot more students, but he'd also limit their access to him.

Several girls gasped and began to cry when Stewart grabbed Jenna's hair and pressed the barrel of the gun hard into her cheek. "What part of *you're not the boss anymore* don't you understand, bitch?"

Mike sprang from his seat and yelled, "Let her go!"

Continuing to hold tight to Jenna's hair, Stewart aimed the gun at him. Mike stopped dead, raised both his hands to his chest, palms facing Stewart, and said in a more controlled voice, "Okay, okay. Let's settle this man to man, Stew."

Like a demon spawned in the center of the sun, anger consumed Stewart as he glared at Mike. Jenna felt the heat of his volatility and braced herself for his violent reaction. With sinister envy, Stewart hissed like a pressure cooker on the verge of exploding. He yelled, "You think you're a man? Are you a tough guy like your fuckin', hot-shot daddy?" He swung his eyes to Jenna then back to Mike. Snorting at him like a bull ready to charge, he laughed sardonically and said, "Okay, big guy. Come here and let Rossi do you like she does your daddy!"

Jenna locked eyes with Mike, but before she could motion for him to sit back down, Stewart threatened, "Now! Or she's dead!"

Stewart yanked Jenna's hair harder and forced her to her knees. Mocking her, he said, "Now, I expect your fuckin' best effort, bitch!"

Despite a combination of fear and anger forcing Mike's body to shake, he lunged at Stewart, but Stewart dodged his attack.

"Try that one more time, junior, and daddy's little toy will have to find a new face." Keeping the gun pointed at Jenna, he ordered Mike, "Let's see what you got, big guy!"

Tears blurred Mike's vision as he wiped his face hard with one hand and dropped his sweat pants to his ankles. Jenna looked up and mouthed, "Stay alive."

Mike stared down at her kneeling at his feet. With one more, quick swipe of his hand across his eyes, he slipped his fingers under the rim of his underwear and wondered how he would ever face his father or her again.

With red-eyed fury, Stewart shouted, "DO IT NOW!"

Tension loomed like a static charge waiting to snap. Some students turned their heads; others closed their eyes and buried their faces in the bend of their arms to stifle their cries.

Suddenly, Caleb Marawski, sitting behind Ken Miller, let loose a high-pitched marauder's laugh. He jumped up with misplaced enthusiasm and said, "This is great, Stew! Before Rossi does Mike, we should have a *Biggest Dong Contest*." He pulled Ken Miller out of his seat, picked him up, and slammed him into the nearby wall. "Let's start with this arrogant prick!"

In the brief time it took an angry Stewart to wave the gun at Caleb and order him to sit down, Caleb whispered to Ken, "His knees on three." With his hands held up high, Caleb turned and shot Stewart a bright, toothy grin and assured him, "I'm on your side, buddy. I can't stand her nagging or this place any more than you can."

Again, Stewart ordered Caleb. "Sit down or I'll blow your dumb Polish head off!"

Jenna sensed an unusual shift in Ken Miller's body language. His back up against the wall, he stood watchful, waiting.

"Hey, Stew, they say you should count when you get mad." Caleb rambled nonsensically saying, "Like *one*, I'm trying to help you get out of this mess alive." He shot Ken a quick glance. "*Two.* If we work together, we can have more fun with all these idiots."

Reminiscent of Friday night under the lights when Ken called the shots, Ken felt the familiar adrenalin rush through his body in anticipation of Caleb's call to take down the opposing force.

That's it, Jenna thought. Caleb's signaling Ken. In a split second, she looked up at Mike and mouthed, "Football."

Like a choreographed dance, a second before Caleb's "*three*," Jenna distracted Stewart with a piercing scream. Ken pushed off the wall and dove low to tackle Stewart at the knees and pull him down. In the same split second, Caleb seized Stewart's hand holding the gun.

Crack! A single bullet discharged from the gun, coursed through Jenna's shoulder, and lodged in a side wall of the room. As Mike pushed Jenna out of the way, Caleb used his head to butt Stewart's face causing blood to spray onto the students sitting in the front row desks. He grabbed Stewart's arm and twisted it until the gun dropped to the floor.

When the initial shock wore off, pandemonium broke loose. Frantic students scrambled toward the door as police rushed in.

Mike cradled Jenna as she bled in his arms. Between sobs, he repeated, "I'm sorry I got him mad. I didn't mean to make things worse."

Before her eyes glazed over and rolled back, she whispered in a barely audible voice, "You're alive."

After the police briefing, Marcus contacted Steve waiting in his car close to the school. "Stewart's in custody. What I know so far is Mike and the kids appear to be fine. Jenna was shot in the shoulder during a scuffle to bring Stew down. Mike and several others are headed for the emergency room with superficial injuries. Give me time to calm the student body and parents lighting up my phone line, and I'll swing by your house tonight."

The Rossis paced the waiting area of the surgical unit as a surgeon worked to repair Jenna's shoulder. In the emergency room, Steve hovered over Mike resting on a gurney as Clare and Tony Gaone sat with the Rossis praying for a positive outcome.

Still dazed by the nightmarish event, Mike's chin shook when he said, "I tried to move her out of the way, Dad." His eyes pooled. "I'm sorry; I'm so sorry."

His one hundred, sixty-pound son morphed into a toddler begging to crawl into the safety of his father's arms. Steve wrapped his arms around his son and felt Mike tremble for several seconds before rallying himself to composure.

Giving him two hard pats on the back, Steve said, "Come on, Mike. Only a fool would second guess any of you in that room. When someone's pointing a gun at you, you do what you need to do to stay alive." He planted a hard, lingering kiss on his head. "You're all alive."

Pushing his head back onto the pillow, Mike's voice was stronger, full of venom. "I swear I'll kill Stewart if I get the chance."

"Stewart has a long, hard row to hoe, Mike. Right now, he's in a world of trouble and may never see daylight."

"Stop feeling sorry for him, Dad. The idiot wanted us to . . ." His voice trailed off as he narrowed his eyes and angrily stared at some distant point in the hallway.

Gripping his son's hand to comfort him, he asked, "Remember what Nonna always says about revenge?"

"Nonna's not always right," he countered with indignation.

"Don't let her hear you say that," he said with levity. "We've been through enough tonight."

Mike mulled his grandmother's mantra. "Revenge is an evil act we choose that robs us of our own goodness." He watched the nurses and doctors scurrying in and out of the emergency cubicles. Voices carrying meaningless messages swirled around him. He swung his eyes laden with skepticism back to his father. "You would've hated both of us, Dad."

With a slight tilt of his head, Steve grabbed Mike's hand, squeezed, and said, "You could be a mass murderer like Charles Manson, and I wouldn't hate you." He threw him a slow, soft punch to the jaw. "Maybe deck you for etching a swastika in your forehead, but hate you? Never!"

The emergency room doctor checked on Mike and confirmed on his clipboard the absence of injuries he concluded earlier.

Mike closed his eyes. His spirit drained; he pleaded, "Can we go home?"

The doctor told Steve, "Give us a half hour, and he can be in his own bed before dark."

Steve gently brushed some strands of hair off Mike's forehead and told him, "I'll be back to get you when they complete the release forms. I'll send Nonna and Pop down here while I check on Jenna."

Keeping his eyes closed, Mike nodded.

"Any word?" Steve asked Dominic Rossi.

Dom wrapped his hands around a white plastic cup and wondered aloud, "What's taking them so long?"

"How's Mike?" Rosie wanted to know.

"Physically, okay. I'm taking him home in a little while." He eyed her apologetically. "I'd like to stay with Jen, but he still feels vulnerable."

"Can you blame him? Those poor kids thought they were going to die today. He needs his father." She gently placed her hand on his cheek and said, "We'll watch over Jenna tonight. You can stand guard in the morning."

Steve's eyes weighed heavily when he said, "Something more than a gun threatened them in that room, Rosie." Worry filled his eyes. "What the hell did that kid make them do?"

Before Rosie could respond, the doctor pushed open the surgical unit doors and announced, "The angels are with us today! The bullet entered and exited Jenna's left shoulder in one clean sweep. We went in, cleaned the wound, and repaired some tissue. There's no major damage." Relief on his face and in his voice, he explained, "Expect some soreness and occasional stiffness for a couple of months. With therapy, she should regain full use of her arm." He repeated, "No doubt about it. God's angels are hovering around here today." Clutching a clipboard to his chest, he told them, "We have her in recovery, sedated, and comfortable. We'll keep her here for a couple of days to guard against infection. She's groggy from the anesthesia, but you'll be able to see her shortly."

Rosie hugged Dom and whispered a prayer of thanksgiving.

Steve dropped in a chair and covered his face with his hands. A whimsical thought played in his mind. He imagined himself Superman speeding through space and time, stopping the earth rotating on its axis. He wanted to steal back time, to change the course of catastrophic events that culminated in those hellish moments in the classroom.

Another family entered the waiting room and jolted him out of his daydream. It was their turn to fret over the well-being of their loved one. Like him, they would have to rely on mere mortal ways to help the person they loved bear the wounds that the dark side of life carved into his body and soul.

The curtains flapped like soft angel-wings as a cool, spring breeze gently streamed through Mike's half-opened window. Feeling confident, he feigned fatigue to convince his hovering father to leave his side. A heavy lonesomeness enveloped him seconds after his father pulled the door almost shut on his way out. Alone now in the dark room, the monotonous sound of beetles droning against the deep purple sky filled him with trepidation. He lay still in his bed and stared uneasily at the single ray of light from the hallway that filtered through the crack of his bedroom door.

His eyes widened at the late knock on the front door. Hugging his pillow close to his chest, he slipped out of bed and stood in the hallway just outside his room.

Downstairs, Steve motioned Marcus in and asked with mild suspicion, "Doesn't your day ever end?"

Marcus rolled his eyes. "I know it's late, but I thought you'd appreciate some insight tonight."

"It had to be bad, Marcus. The last time I saw Mike cry like this, he was facing down a bully in a sandbox." Confused, Steve said, "First he's edgy and apologetic; then he hides behind this bravado, like nothing out of the ordinary happened today."

Mike slowly slid down the wall, sat on the floor, and buried his face in the pillow he was holding. He's going to find out, he thought. Breathing heavily into the pillow, he strained to listen as flashbacks of another late-night conversation chilled him to the bone. He remembered the same helpless feeling that engulfed him when he overheard his grandmother consoling his father over his mother's impending death.

Marcus told Steve, "Right now that classroom's a crime scene. The police need a few days to gather evidence, then we'll call the students back. Trauma counselors will be available. I want these kids and the community to understand that we won't let fear shut us down. We instructed the faculty to let the administrators deal with the media."

"Why won't anyone talk about what really happened in that room, Marcus?"

Marcus held up his hand, palm facing Steve, and said, "No matter what it sounds like, keep in mind, they're all alive."

Steve placed his hand on his chest and said in earnest, "I love my son more than anything or anyone in this world. I'm not about to play Monday morning quarterback on what went down."

Mike raised his head, breathed a deep sigh of relief, and strained to listen.

"Stewart planned to herd the students into a corner and kill as many of them as he could." Marcus ran his hand through his hair before saying, "First, Jenna forced a showdown when she foiled his plan by ordering the kids to sit back down. Enraged, Stewart shoved the gun into her face. Then Mike forced another showdown when he jumped up to defend her. That's when it became personal between Stewart and Mike."

Steve covered his face and said, "Good God, he tried to be a hero."

Marcus nodded saying, "By all accounts, the kids insist he was one of the heroes."

Feeling flush, Mike sat in the hallway thinking: Nothing like a half-naked hero for the school to talk about for the rest of my life.

Marcus said, "In Stewart's prehistoric brain, Mike challenged his manhood. Manhood to these kids equals sex." He sank back on the couch and paused a longer time searching for tasteful words to disclose the obscene activity that came close to happening.

Steve winced asking, "So Mike's twisted up inside because he had to engage in sex to stay alive?"

Mike sat up, frozen. He held his breath and listened to the squalid details Marcus described.

Marcus decided that being direct was the best way to clear the air and ease the anxiety of his friend. "Stewart insisted that Jenna perform oral sex on Mike."

Steve's jaw dropped, followed quickly with an incredulous, "What?"

Marcus held up his hand and said emphatically, "It never happened, Steve!" He stood and asked, "Do you have any vodka?"

Using his index finger to stir the ice in his drink, Marcus said in mild disbelief, "Of all the kids on the planet, Caleb Marawski jumps up and calls a football play." He shook his head in wonderment. "Every kid in that class testified someone would have died today if Caleb, Mike, and Kenny didn't take Stewart down."

Steve's eyes shifted in the direction of the stairs. "That's why he keeps apologizing. He believes I'll hold what almost happened with Jenna against him."

Marcus nodded. "Before we pray for mass amnesia, we all need to remember that those kids prevented a tragedy." Opening the door to leave, he turned, and said, "If a hostage situation can happen in Sparta, it can happen anywhere in this country." His eyes tired and his face worn, he added, "I know we can't reach every wounded, seething soul, but when we don't, look at the colossal pain and damage one angry person can inflict on humanity at the drop of a dime. God only knows how many funerals we'd be planning this week if Jenna and those boys didn't act smart and courageous."

Steve switched off the lights and climbed the stairs. Rounding the corner, he spotted Mike sitting on the hallway floor staring up at him.

"Did you hear everything Dr. Wright had to say?"

Mike nodded sheepishly.

Sitting Indian style facing his son, he asked, "Was Marcus's account accurate?"

"Pretty much."

"Did he skip over anything important?"

Mike's eyes watered. "She would've done it to save us, Dad."

Steve tilted his head and studied his son's face. "Do you believe any part of this ordeal is your fault?"

Mike shrugged.

Steve's head fell; his chin rested on his chest. Several seconds passed before he looked up and said, "Maybe it's my fault, Mike. I should've waited until you graduated before getting involved with Jenna." Continuing to eye him, he said, "Maybe Stewart retaliated against you because I verbally slam-dunked his father in front of him at the sportsmen's extravaganza."

Mike sat silent, fixing his eyes on an old stain on the hallway carpet.

"Then again, maybe it's not your fault or my fault. Maybe it's Jenna's fault."

Mike looked up. "How's it her fault?"

"Think about it. Stewart hated her. She was bossy. She called him out for stealing the water at the sportsmen's event." He paused for several moments before saying, "It could be Ahmad's fault. Isn't he the one who started the rumor that Jenna was going to fail Stewart, stop him from graduating?"

A slight grin formed on Mike's mouth. "Man, Nonna would have a field day if she heard us talking about who's to blame."

Steve let out a short laugh. "The lady calls 'em as she sees 'em." He reached over and brushed Mike's hair back. "How would Nonna call this one?"

"She already told me, 'Stewart Jones came with the gun. He's the one responsible.'"

Steve stood and reached for Mike's hand to help him up. Mike's eyes pooled when he said, "She was kneeling at my feet, Dad. She would've . . ." He closed his eyes to force back the tears.

Steve drew his muscular son into his arms. "I know it was bad, Mike, but all things considered, it's a pretty good day."

Mike broke from his father's embrace. Surprise mixed with wonder, he asked, "How can you possibly find anything good about today, Dad? It's almost as bad as the day Mom died."

"I wish I had the power to turn back the clock for you, Mike, but I don't. So, while I've been sorting through this mess, I found out my son helped save a lot of lives, and the woman I love loves me enough to do whatever it takes to keep the most important person in my life alive. I'd say we all did a superb job of keeping the water outta the ship today."

Mike bit his bottom lip and nodded. Wiping the mist from his eyes with his fingers, he said, "Nonna's coming tomorrow morning, but I'd like to go to the hospital in the afternoon." Before heading to bed, he said, "Maybe I'll get some of the guys to tag along."

Steve nodded, grabbed his son's face, and planted a firm kiss on his forehead. "You're one smart, tough kid."

Mike shrugged. "One second I feel like I can leap tall buildings with a single bound; the next second, my teeth are clattering under my blanket like a two-year-old who needs my daddy to tuck me in."

"Sounds normal after a life-death situation. The sooner you get back to your routine, the more confident you'll feel in your ability to control your surroundings." He picked up the pillow lying on the floor and tossed it to Mike. "Soon enough, you won't be needing your daddy around."

Pushing the door open to his room, Mike turned to his father and said, "But I'll always want you around."

The sun broke through the narrow crack in the hospital curtains that didn't quite lock together at the center. Keeping vigil over Jenna, Dom and Rosie were sitting in a pair of yellow, leather chairs, when Steve walked into the room.

He wrapped his arms around Rosie and said, "Go catch breakfast. I'll call you when she wakes."

Not long after, the clatter of breakfast trays being delivered to patients up and down the hall awakened Jenna. Blinking several times, she slowly surveyed the room and settled on Steve's familiar face. Panic seized her when she had flashbacks of Stewart Jones holding the gun to her head.

Sweating profusely, she struggled to sit up and asked, "Did he hurt Mike?"

Sitting on the edge of the bed, Steve calmed her. "Mike's safe. All the kids are fine." He smiled down at her and said, "Rumor has it a posse's arriving at high noon. I figured you'd want help combing your hair and slapping on some makeup like the superficial, self-centered creature you've shown yourself to be."

She let out a weak laugh. Seconds later, she closed her eyes to stop hot tears from rolling onto her cheeks.

He placed a tissue in her hand and whispered, "It's over. Everyone's safe."

Keeping her eyes clamped shut; she gave a quick shake of her head. "Do you know what he wanted us . . ." She turned her face from him.

"Mike and Marcus gave me an account."

"He planned to kill us."

Sitting on the side of her bed, he massaged her hand and said, "I had this conversation with Mike last night. He's bombarded with the same feelings of fear, embarrassment, and guilt that you're probably feeling." Canvassing her face, he said, "You and those boys prevented a massacre." Gently tapping her chest with his index finger, he said, "The only thing left to do now is to let Caleb hear you tell him he has character."

She whispered Caleb's name with an air of whimsy. Her eyes grew large and her body animated recalling, "At first I thought he joined Stewart. He hoisted Kenny out of his seat like he was picking up a rag doll. It all happened so fast." Her eyes narrowed as she pondered before saying, "Something about Kenny's face was off. He didn't look scared, like a kid being bullied in front of his peers. He looked ready, waiting for something to happen." Unable to control her excitement, she tried to lift her arms to demonstrate how Mike shoved her out of the way.

"Ouch!" she said, wincing.

"Keep still, Jen. They just patched you up a few hours ago."

As he fluffed her pillows and raised the bed so she could rest comfortably in a seated position, she told him, "We all have to go back to school as soon as possible. I don't want fear to settle in."

"The school plans to open in a few days." Handing her a glass of water with a straw, he said, "Talk about it with the boys today. Making plans will give them a sense of future."

Before she could respond, her phone rang.

His face sagged when he heard a voice whisper, "I need Jenna."

He pressed mute and said, "It's Sam. I'll tell her you're resting."

Motioning for him to give her the phone, she mustered exuberance and said, "Hi, Sam!"

As if a noose restricting the air that she breathed loosened, Samantha Kind blurted out, "Thank God you're alive!" before she broke into heavy sobs.

"Stop the drama, Sam. I'm okay." She winked at Steve and told her, "I have a wound to my shoulder is all. I'll be home tomorrow, and with some therapy, I'll be as good as new."

"It's all coming back, Jen. Remembering what they did to me is so" her voice barely audible when she whispered, "hard." Catching Jenna off guard, she yelled, "What kind of parents force their kid to watch them beat each other up and then have sex?"

Steve cocked his head, frowned, and motioned for Jenna to hang up.

Jenna mouthed, "Ten minutes."

"Your parents were ill, Sam. They never got help, but you're getting the help you need. You'll be stronger and better, and you'll love your children."

"Oooh" she said with determination. "I will never allow this to happen to another child. Never!" After several hard sniffles she said, "They didn't love me. Your mom was the only one who ever made me feel special." Her voice transitioned to toddler mode saying, "She cooked me angel hair pasta cuz . . . cuz I was . . . I was her angel." Reasoning more like an adult, she asked, "How can I ever have kids when I'm so afraid to . . ." More clinical, she said, "People can't get better without someone who believes in them. Tell me you believe I'll get better, Jen." Before Jenna could respond, Sam said, "Sometimes I feel like killing myself, but," her voice fell into a whisper, "it scares me cuz I'd like to take a lot of other people with me." A glass clinked as she filled it with liquor to dull her pain. Rambling, she said, "There're crazier people out there than me. I never tried ta kill anyone like that jackass kid in your class. My father doesn't count cuz he wanted ta kill me." With more vehemence, she yelled, "They should cut off that kid's hands. That'll teach'em. Lock his baby ass up in jail." A guttural groan released the pain that welled in her aching heart. "People probably love him more than anyone ever loved me."

Steve looked at Jenna, and said louder than he should have, "Her drunken tirade's not helping you."

Jenna covered the phone and whispered, "She's almost done." To Sam, she said, "We love you, Sam, and I'll always be here for you."

Relief poured from her. "Thaaank you, Jen. I needed ta hear it." She whimpered, "I was always a good little girl." Her voice carried resentment when she said, "People act like it's my fault I lost my job. Like I made myself sick. My doctor says my body remembers all the horrible abuse even though I can't remember most of what they did to me. It was really bad." After a short pause and some deeper breaths, she said more confidently, "I'm doing the best I can. I clean my house, pay my bills, take care of my car, make my appointments. God, what else do people want from me? You have a father that never screwed you and a boyfriend that does, so where do you get off telling me I should be doing more?"

"We only want to help you be happy, Sam."

She let out a long groan before saying, "I know you do. I'm sorry I yelled." Mimicking a child, she said, "I wuv you."

"I love you, too, Sam."

Drowning in liquor, her child-like voice garbled, "Okay, I'mtirednow. I'll slip in by med . . . I mean my bed now. Do you wuv me, Jen?"

"I wuv you, Sam."

"I know you do," she said, laughing. Then she chastised Jenna with, "Stop talking like a baby. I hope they lock that kid up forever for shootin' you."

"Get some rest, Sam. I'll talk to you tomorrow."

Making little attempt to hide his irritation, Steve told Jenna, "I'm beginning to believe you have a masochistic streak in you."

Growing eerily quiet, a vision came to Jenna. A whimpering Samantha lay in her crib. Desiring comfort, the child stares at her emotionally disturbed mother emptied of all nurturing qualities. The mother shoves a pacifier into Sam's mouth and presses down hard. Sam lets out one weak whimper and slips into safer oblivion.

"Jenna?"

After a hard blink, she stared at Steve.

"She abuses you, Jen."

"No, Stephen. Stop getting it wrong. I'm not the victim. Sam's always been the victim."

"What makes you think your misplaced guilt can make her well?" he countered with a vehement whisper. "Get it through your head that she's never going to be normal."

Her tired eyes widened. "Does hope only belong to the normal? Are you normal? Am I? Look at us. We've experienced love all our lives, and we still struggle to trust." She sighed saying, "I used to laugh at my grandfather when he'd say, 'Keep the water outta the ship.'" Weak but defiant, she told him, "All Sam's life, she's been reduced to begging for crumbs of sympathy from people. Who helps her keep the water outta the ship?"

Deflecting traces of remorse, Steve said, "Maybe if Sam wasn't so preoccupied with transforming trauma into an art, people might be more willing to pick up a pail and help her bail some water."

Feeling the strain of her shoulder wound and the emotional struggle with Steve, her voice was tired and more conciliatory. "Because of one horrible experience with a guy in college, it took me over ten years to trust a man again. Imagine what I'd be like if I had to swallow my father's garbage every day." Her eyes fell as she picked at her blanket. "If Mike and I would've . . ." Looking up, she asked, "How is Mike?"

"He gets clammy at the drop of a hat, but that's to be expected after the kind of trauma he experienced."

She dabbed her eyes with the corner of the bed sheet and asked, "You think so?"

Bothered by her sarcasm, he said, "What happened defies sensibilities. It's not unreasonable to think all of you, including Mike, will need a lot of assurance to get back on track."

Her voice softened; her sympathetic eyes appealed to his reason. "If Mike needs assurance because he experienced an isolated trauma, how much assurance do you think he'd need if Stewart would've succeeded?"

The color drained from Steve's face. Reluctantly nodding agreement, he asked, "We're not talking only about Mike, are we?"

Jenna choked back tears.

Handing her a tissue, he asked, "Did they really hurt Sam as much as she claims?"

"Whatever those monsters did, they succeeded in creating an emotionally deficient thirty-three-year-old struggling to find someone to affirm her worth." More reflective, she said, "You and friends like Myra can't understand why I care so much about her. We howl when we remember the stunned look on her face, how she was petrified of that guy at the ballpark threatening to shove a footlong down her throat." Swallowing hard, she said, "I guess shoving a six-inch penis down a kid's throat will conjure that kind of horrible reaction." More resolved, she said, "All Sam ever dreamed was to have my life, not a movie star's life, or some other famous person's life, but *my* life." Idling in sadness, she said, "The least I can do is share myself with her and try to be a friend who helps her to understand that she isn't the sum of what her parents did to her."

Pecking her cheek, he teased saying, "Okay, I get it. Just tell me I don't have to get close enough for her to chop off my six inch—"

Jenna let out a weak laugh. "Sam imagines you're twelve inches long, but no matter what she threatens, male genitalia are to her what sunlight is to a vampire. But just in case," she winked, "I can love a physical eunuch. It's the moral eunuchs I find repulsive."

Raising his brow, he said with mock appreciation, "That certainly allays my fears." Still skeptical, he asked, "Could she be exaggerating her experiences?"

"Even if you discount half her stories, they never held her with tenderness, never planted kisses on her face, and never sang *Happy Birthday* to her."

Fighting the melancholic spirit threatening to fill the room, he pulled her breakfast tray across the bed, and said, "You better eat before the eggs get cold."

She shook her head. "I'd rather feel your arms around me while I close my eyes and rest."

"My pleasure," he told her as he rolled the breakfast tray aside and gently laid his head on her chest, careful not to add pressure to her bandaged shoulder. She drifted off as the soft, steady beat of her heart widened his compassion.

A half hour passed before two detectives knocked on Jenna's door hoping to ask her more questions about the hostage situation that unfolded in her room the day before.

Holding her hand, Steve asked, "Are you up to talking about it one more time?"

Jenna nodded saying, "Talking about it may be easier than harboring it for the rest of our lives."

That Friday, the police department, school officials, and key students involved in the crisis held a joint news conference to quell the misinformation circulating throughout the community. Local news as well as national news affiliates pressed the panel for details.

While most of the questions were benign, an accusatory reporter singled out Marcus Wright and asked, "According to my sources, the school suspended the alleged gunman for sexual harassment of Miss Rossi that took place at a gun show in the school only weeks prior to the takeover. Was it wise for school officials to permit the student to re-enter the school, especially Miss Rossi's classroom?"

With an edge to his voice, Marcus first defended the *Sportsmen's Gun and Game Extravaganza* by saying, "We've coordinated the annual sportsmen's event for decades. The gun show you're referring to is more a gun display, and it's a small part of what this community learning experience offers. We make sure qualified instructors teach a healthy respect for various kinds of weapons: guns, knives, bows." Addressing the second part of the reporter's question with equal confidence, Marcus said, "If we permanently barred from school every student who spoke or acted inappropriately, our schools would be empty. Our knowledgeable and caring guidance department constantly works with our teachers to design individualized programs to help *at risk* students meet the requirements for graduation." There was unmistakable defiance in Marcus's eyes when he ended saying, "That's what we do, sir. We help every student, even the troubled ones." His eyes swung to Jenna. "Miss Rossi was collecting research paper revisions. Stewart Jones was legally in school. He was following all the rules up until the moment he allegedly pulled out a gun that had no connection with the school's sportsmen's event."

The chief of police called on one last reporter. Addressing Mike Goane, the reporter asked, "What were your thoughts when you were seconds away from having sex with your teacher in front of your classmates?"

Jenna's mouth gaped at the same time Marcus jumped up in protest. Steve signaled his son not to answer the question. Taking them by surprise, Mike raised his hand to quiet the crowd.

"I'll give you an answer, but you won't like it any more than any of us like that question." With more composure than he thought he possessed, Mike said, "I'm glad Kenny and Caleb were in the room with me instead of you. They only had seconds to decide to make their choices count. You had days to choose a good question, and all you thought about was sex." Glancing back at Jenna, he said, "Miss Rossi's a good teacher, but she lectures us a lot."

Soft laughter rippled through the room as Jenna palmed her face to hide her embarrassment.

"She even printed the word *character* in big bold letters on the board to remind us that without character, everything else falls short." He pointed at Caleb and said, "We're writing his name next to that word when we go back to school."

The room erupted in applause.

Ken blurted out, "How about *Brave New World*?"

From his place in the room, Steve folded his arms over his chest and nodded acknowledgment of the familiar Rossi rant.

Mike explained, "One day someone complained about homework, and Miss Rossi went off on us about *Brave New World*. She warned how a handful of leaders will control every part of our lives if we don't arm ourselves with knowledge." He raised his brows and said, "I guess it's easier for governments to control dumb people. That's why dictators burn books, and slaves were forbidden to read and write." He eyed the reporter and said, "You guys should sit in on her freedom lecture. Freedom of religion, the right to bear arms, and the right to assemble are all important, but if you reporters aren't willing to ask the right questions, investigate, and use facts, then we can kiss all the other freedoms good-bye." Surveying the room, he asked, "If reporters don't highlight what's important, what are we supposed to research when we want to make good decisions?" Pointing to Caleb, he said, "You could've asked him what motivated him to jump up and call a play to save our lives when Stewart was waving a gun in his face." Pointing to Ken, he said, "You could've asked him what he was thinking when Caleb picked him up and positioned him for the play to tackle Stewart. How about asking Miss Rossi what she was thinking when she stopped Stewart from herding us into a corner?"

Silence loomed heavily in the room before Mike said, "People across the country will read the articles that you write about us. What's more important, the sex that almost happened, or the courage everyone displayed?" After biting his bottom lip for several seconds, he admitted, "We were all scared, but we kept each other alive. We even kept Stewart alive." With a friendlier tone, he addressed the reporter, and said, "We'll find out what you believe is important when we read tomorrow's paper and check out what's trending on Twitter."

The packed room met the heartrending condemnation of the reporter's question with sustained applause. Caleb stood and draped his arm across Mike's shoulders. Within seconds, Ken flanked him on the other side. With insatiable fervor, photographers snapped photos of the trio. They motioned for Jenna to join them.

The next day, headlines across the country read, *Courage Kept Spartan Students Alive.*

Chapter Fourteen

Swirling clouds dipped low as Frank McCoy rounded the bend on his routine morning run through a suburb of Waldorf, Maryland. In a nick of time, he yanked the newspaper from its cylinder case, sprinted to the back door, and dashed inside before the heavens opened up and let loose a torrential rain. He grabbed a bottle of water, flipped open the paper, and dropped it on the kitchen counter. The caption beneath the photo spread across the front page drained his face of color. Holding the edge of the counter to steady himself, he eased onto a stool. The soft clicking of his wife's heels as she moved down the hallway and entered the kitchen prompted him to composure.

Fastening her bracelet, Kim McCoy complained, "Of all the days for it to pour. I hope it clears up for the rummage sale."

Frank sat silent, his eyes glued to the front page.

Looking up, she asked, "What's wrong, hon?"

He slid the paper across the counter and said, "I can't believe it's her."

Kim covered her face with her hands and let out a soft gasp. "It is her! We need to contact her right now, I mean right this minute." She reached for the phone, but her husband blocked her hand.

"We can't do that, Kim. She has to contact us."

"What about Carly? She doesn't have all the time in the world to wait for Jenna Rossi to feel like getting in touch with her." She stared at the newspaper. "What if she would have been killed?"

"She's very much alive, and we can't afford to get embroiled in bureaucratic red tape that lands Carly in a foster home. We can live without the extra financial and emotional hassles right now, too."

Kim's soft voice shook with emotion. "How much longer can we wait?"

Frank stared at Jenna's picture before noticing Carly holding onto the banister as she robotically descended the stairs.

"How you feel today, princess?"

"Better than yesterday," she said, sitting on the bottom step to catch her breath. "What're you arguing about now?"

Kim stared down at the frail teen and asked, "Did you hear about the latest school hostage crisis?"

Taking a deep breath, she said, "I haven't felt like getting online for a few days." Pointing to the paper in Kim's hands, she asked, "Is that story about them?"

Kim nodded. She eyed her husband with contrite defiance as she handed Carly the paper.

"Oh my gosh! That teacher could be my twin."

Frank let out a sarcastic laugh.

"You don't think I was a twin, and the nuns separated us at birth?"

"No, Carly, you're a one and only. Besides, that teacher's old enough to be your mother."

Carly stared at Jenna's picture. "What are the chances this lady went to France and had a baby?" Rolling her eyes, she tossed the paper onto the floor, and said, "After everything she's been through, I bet she'd love to hear someone like me say, 'Hi, I'm Carly McCoy. You might be my mother. Can I have a hug before I die?'"

Tired of masking her broken heart, Carly bent her head down to her knees and sobbed. Kim squeezed beside her on the step and draped her arm across her daughter's shoulders.

"Are you going to cry about it, or do something about it?"

Carly looked up with hot tears stinging her eyes. "What am I supposed to do, Mom? Look at me. I'm half dead."

Kim grabbed Carly's mouth and planted a kiss on it. "This smart mouth tells me you're very much alive." Hugging her, she urged, "You can sit around like an old log waiting to be tossed on the fire, or you can use every breath God gives you to accomplish some goals."

Frank shot his wife a cold stare. "Stop right now, Kim. Can't you see she's tired? Once this genie's out of the bottle—"

Kim blurted out a curt, "No!" Standing, she added, "Carly's waited long enough. It's not about us. It's not about Jenna Rossi, and it's not even about the law." A wave of sympathy for Carly swept over her when she said, "This child wants to feel her mother's arms around her one time, and we're going to help her do that right now!" She narrowed her eyes and threatened with deadly determination. "Jenna Rossi's going to hug Carly if I have to hold her hostage myself!"

Carly's eyes bulged. Swinging her eyes to Frank, she asked, "You really think this lady's my mother?"

Emotionally aligned with his wife, Frank let out a deep sigh. "We know she's your mother. I just don't want any legal problems, and I don't want you disappointed." Staring at Kim, he said, "You were in the room when Sister Martine warned us not to contact her."

Hope danced in Carly's eyes. "What if a dying kid searching for her mother decided to contact a lady who looked like she could be her long-lost mother?"

Frank crossed his arms over his chest and said, "Something tells me we're about to find out." Eyeing Carly with concern, he asked, "What if she doesn't want to meet with you? She could be a self-centered chick who runs from responsibilities." He reached down for Carly's hand and pulled her into his arms. "Do you want to live with that knowledge, princess?"

She buried her face in his chest. "You're my mother and father. I love you with all my heart." Looking up at him, she added, "Yeah, it'll suck if she doesn't want to see me, but at least I'll know I tried."

Kim wrapped her arms around them. She glanced down at Jenna's picture with Mike, Caleb, and Kenny flanking her.

"She won't reject you, baby. That lady has a good heart."

"And you know that how?" Frank asked.

"She could have easily had an abortion, but she didn't. She was willing to compromise herself to save a classroom full of kids." Her eyes pierced Jenna's picture. "There's strength in her, and Carly inherited her strength." She kissed Carly's bare head. "I wouldn't be surprised if she needs to feel *your* arms around her just as much as you need *her* arms around you."

Unable to contain her excitement. Carly asked, "Can I call her now?"

"Hold up," Frank cautioned. "If we can't stop you from going rogue, at least give the lady a couple of days to recuperate before she has to deal with a force named Carly McCoy."

Chapter Fifteen

LOUNGING ON HER SOFA ON A LAZY SUNDAY AFTERNOON, Jenna caressed Steve's arm, and said, "Chaperone the bon-fire with me. The kids love when you're around."

"I'll let you know by the middle of the week."

She sat up and drew her knees to her chest. "This has been one, long, exhausting month." With one hand holding her hair back into a pony tail, she let out a deep sigh, and said, "I guess Stewart will spend time in prison, but at least he'll get the counseling he needs." After a pause she added, "I'll be relieved when Patsy Zarone walks across the stage, tucks his diploma under his arm, and we all go home."

Checking some upcoming appointments on his phone, he said, "These kids will be telling their grandchildren what happened in this school."

"We did okay, didn't we?"

Tucking his phone into his shirt pocket, he said, "The students, the community kept the water out of the ship."

Jenna said, "Speaking of dry ships, I can go for a cold bottle of water."

Standing to stretch his legs, he said, "Coming up."

On his way to the refrigerator, the blinking red light on Jenna's answering machine caught Steve's eye.

"When's the last time you checked your messages, Jen?"

"Last night," she said, through a wide yawn.

"Someone wants your attention."

"Probably another reporter," she moaned. "See who it is."

He pressed play on his way to handing her the water. A youthful voice started unsure, then grew in excitement.

"Hi! I hope. . . I hope Jenna Rossi gets this message. My name is Carly McCoy. I . . . I live in Waldorf, Maryland. I saw your picture in the newspaper. I'm happy you're safe. I want you to know that I'm a fourteen-year-old girl who was born in a convent in France. I'm dying to hug you and say thank you. Please call me at this number if . . . if you want to talk to me as much as I've dreamed of talking to you."

Jenna dropped the bottle of water and covered her gaping mouth with her hands. "That's her! My baby found me!" She jumped up and flew to the answering machine. Hugging the machine to her chest, she kept pressing play to listen to Carly's voice over and over again. "She's dying to hug me, Steve. She's dying to hug me!" Grabbing the phone, she began to dial Carly's number.

"Hold on, Jen." Corralling her in his arms, he said, "Think this through for a moment. Her parents may not know she contacted you. There may be legalities."

Jenna wilted in his arms. "How do I let her know I've spent fourteen years longing to hug her, too?"

Steve guided her back to the couch where they considered several scenarios.

"I'll contact Carly and tell her I need to talk to her parents before we move to the next step. I won't mention your name."

"What if she's not on good terms with her parents?"

"All the more reason we need to move carefully," he convinced her. "Let's avoid wading into a family mess."

"When will you call?"

Holding up his phone, he asked with a tease, "Is right now fast enough for you?"

"Oh my gosh! I can't believe this is really happening."

He held his index finger to his lips and said, "Shhh. It's ringing."

"Hi, this is Carly. I can't come to the phone right now, but if you leave your name and credit card number, I'll get back to you after my shopping spree."

Her greeting generated a broad smile. He left a cryptic message ending with, "What would be ideal is if you ask your parents to be available for discussion when you return this phone call."

"What if we scare her away, Steve?"

Chuckling, he said, "That greeting's from a gutsy kid. That article told her where you work, and she knows your name and phone number. You'll be seeing Ms. Carly McCoy sooner than you think."

The advent of being reunited with her child electrified every fiber in her body. "I can hardly breathe. If she doesn't call soon I'll—"

The ring tone of Steve's phone cut her breath off.

"Where are you, Mike?"

Jenna rolled her hands to urge a quick end to the call.

Steve held up his hand to calm her. "Sounds like a plan. See you tonight. Have your work done."

He motioned for Jenna to come closer and said, "Her call came in hours ago. Right now, she may be in an area where there are no towers, so you may be waiting for hours, maybe days."

Jenna sat on his lap and said, "Hold me before I crumble to pieces."

He was massaging her back when the phone made her jump up. Holding her breath, she watched Steve's eyes brighten.

"Hi, this is Carly McCoy. May I . . . May I speak to Mr. Gaone?"

"Speaking. Before we go any further, Carly, may I speak to your parents?"

Carly handed the phone to her mother. There was unmistakable excitement in Kim McCoy's voice when she said, "Mr. Gaone, I'm Carly's mother. My husband, Frank, is standing here with us. Do I have your consent to use the speaker phone so we all can participate in the conversation?"

"Of course."

Steve kept his eyes on Jenna now kneeling in front of him. While she waited for him to signal the okay to connect with the lost part of her soul, he kept her out of the discussion until he knew better in which direction the events would lead.

"Are you aware that Carly made the initial phone call to Jenna Rossi's answering machine?"

Frank answered, "Yes, we know what she did."

Steve said, "There's interest on this end to fulfill her request, but we're not sure if legalities are involved."

Frank said, "We only know that Sister Martine warned us not to contact Jenna Rossi. Carly managed to do that on her own after reading the article about the Spartan hostage crisis."

"For clarification," Steve countered, "do you want this meeting to take place between your daughter and her biological mother?"

"We do. We'd also like to explain our determination for this meeting. If Jenna Rossi is listening, we can assure her that she's legally safe. We will attest that Carly made the initial call. We in no way mean to threaten her or insert ourselves in her life if she desires to remain unavailable." Frank's voice cracked. "I'll be honest with you, Mr. Gaone. Carly doesn't have much—"

"No, Frank! What if they take her away?" Kim blurted out.

"Mr. and Mrs. McCoy, I promise you Jenna Rossi only wants to know that Carly is loved and thriving."

Frank cleared his throat and swallowed hard before continuing. "We love Carly more than our own lives, but she's been battling leukemia for two years. She's worn out." His voice shook. "All she wants now, all we can give her is to know her biological mother loved her. She wants . . ." Choking up, he held Carly and brushed his cheek on her bare head.

"All she wants is a hug from her mother," Kim completed her husband's thought. "Carly contacted Jenna Rossi with our blessing." There was silence on both ends until Kim asked, "Will she do that for Carly? She loved her enough to give her life. We pray that she loves her enough to make our baby's wish come true."

Steve locked eyes with Jenna. His mind raced. What words could he use to tell her that her child was dying? His voice soft and low, he asked, "First, may I explain these circumstances to Jenna?"

"Is Jenna Rossi with you right now?"

"Yes, but—"

"Believe me, Mr. Gaone; I fully understand," Kim said, sympathetically. "We've been living with the grief for some time. Finally, to find your child then learn you'll lose her forever will be devastating."

"Thank you," he said. In a forced upbeat tone, he asked, "Carly?"

"I'm here," she said with a hopeful tone.

"I'm going to hand the phone to Jenna Rossi."

Jenna gripped the phone. Her voice breathless and shaking, she said, "Hi Carly. I love you, and I love your name. I love your voice. Not a day goes by that I don't love you and say a prayer for you. I even have a Christmas tree with all kinds of decorations—"

"Oh my gosh!" Carly squealed. "I can't believe I'm talking to you!" She covered her mouth with her hands and jumped up and down. She hugged her dad. "Mom was so right!" She turned toward the phone. "You sound like an angel."

Jenna cried and said, "I can't wait to hold you, and kiss you, and tell you all about—"

"When can you come? This week? Even if it's spring, can I decorate the Christmas tree with you? Puhleeze, please say you'll come."

"Mr. and Mrs. McCoy, whatever's convenient for you."

"Is this Friday too soon?" Kim asked, minimizing the possibility of second thoughts or a physical setback pre-empting Carly's dream.

Jenna mouthed, "This Friday?" to Steve.

Steve held up his thumb.

"Mr. and Mrs. McCoy?"

"We're here," Kim said.

"I don't mean to sound presumptuous, but, my mother and father have lived with a gaping hole in their hearts because I never gave them a chance to hold . . ." She choked up. Composing herself quickly, she continued, "Carly's their only grandchild, and they've longed to know she's safe, that she's with good parents who love her."

The McCoys asked Carly, "What do you think, sweetheart? Can you handle a family reunion?"

Carly squealed, "This is so unreal! I can't wait to hug all of you!"

Kim McCoy said, "The entire Rossi clan probably heard Carly's answer."

Exiting speaker phone, Kim asked Jenna, "May I have a private word with you?"

Drying her eyes with the bottom edge of her jersey, Jenna said, "Of course."

"I don't know what your circumstances were fourteen years ago, or why you traveled across an ocean to have your baby. All I know is from the moment Sister Martine placed Carly in my arms, each day I've asked God to grace you with every good thing in life. You could have easily discarded this beautiful child. Instead, you gifted us with the light and love of our lives."

Her heart overflowing with appreciation and joy, Jenna said, "Thank you for loving her better than . . ." She let out a soft cry.

"I don't know about better," Kim mused. "Only one certainty exists. I remind Carly from time to time that Frank and I wouldn't have been able to love her with all our hearts if you didn't love her first."

Jenna covered her mouth with her hands and said, "I can't believe I'm going to hold my baby this Friday." Standing, she said, "My parents will finally get to hold her and know she's happy and safe." She threw up her arms, danced in a circle, and squealed, "I'm so happy!" She grabbed Steve's face and kissed him hard. "Thank you for being here, for sharing this magical moment."

His sober response to her excitement gave her pause.

"What?"

Biting down hard on his bottom lip, he looked off to the side and blinked back tears.

She knelt in front of him, cupped his face, and forced him to look at her.

Her stomach knotting, she said, "Tell me, Steve."

"She's sick, Jen."

Jenna pulled back, stood, and asked with an edge to her voice, "How sick?"

Steve gave his head a slow, futile shake.

Clamping her eyes shut, Jenna crossed her arms over her chest. Silence stifled the room as the joy seeped out of her. Seconds later, a primal groan released the pain that welled deep within her. Like a prize fighter weakening after dancing around the ring for fourteen rounds of intense pummeling, this final hard right to her spirit forced her to her knees.

"I can't do this. I can't lose her again."

"Come on, Jen."

Kneeling in stone silence, her eyes glazed over, lifeless. Several moments passed before she looked up and asked, "Why?" Drained of all purpose, she bent her head down to the floor, buried her face in her hands, and sobbed.

Understanding her world turned upside down, the only thing Steve could do was drop to the floor, hold her close, and allow her to run out of tears.

Lying listless in his arms, he gave her a gentle shake, and asked, "What would you tell me if I just learned Mike was going to die?"

"Mike always knew you loved him," her robotic voice countered.

Holding her face, he said, "So, it's the *knowing* that's important. Carly's been fighting to live long enough to know your love and let you know she loves you."

The slight smile that formed on his face prompted her to say, "God can't even spin this one, Stephen."

Caressing her cheek, he said, "I was picturing Carly dancing and squealing when she heard your mom and dad were coming to dinner with us. She reminded me of you jumping around on the dock when I was battling that largemouth bass." He said more seriously, "Someone could live a hundred years and never experience a profound moment. Today, you made Carly the happiest girl in the world, and Friday, you'll cradle her in your arms." He tilted his head and shot her a half-smile to encourage her to fight the flood of despair threatening to pull her under.

"Now what?" she asked.

"Remember our first date? You asked me to teach you everything I know."

She grabbed a pillow lying on the floor and angrily tossed it on the couch. "I asked you to teach me half of what you know," she corrected him.

"Yeah, but you've been teaching me more than I teach you."

Wiping her eyes with her hands, her tone was more resigned. "You taught me how to camp."

"No doubt an important activity," he said, winking. "More important than camping, we're both being reminded that the quality of life isn't measured by time; it's measured by love. I used to fear uncertainty. After Amy died, my mother taught Mike and me that we'd benefit more, grow stronger, if we took chances on friendships and love."

She melted into his arms and cried, "I don't want her to die."

"We can't stop her death, Jen, but we can be a joyful part of the rest of her life."

"Now I know how Prince Hector felt going into battle. The gods tricked him into believing he could actually win for a change." She wiped her face hard with her hands. "We all delude ourselves into thinking God's on our side." Reaching for her keys, she said, "Let's go tell my mom and dad they have a date with their granddaughter." She closed her eyes to stop another onslaught of tears. "Then I'll tell them to prepare for her funeral."

"What a pleasant surprise," Rosie sang out as Jenna and Steve entered the kitchen.

Shrugging off her mother's enthusiasm, Jenna asked, "Where's Dad?"

"Right here," Dom announced as he emerged from the basement. Dusting off his hands, he hugged Jenna, and extended his hand to Steve. Eyeing Jenna, he said, "You look tired, princess. Everything okay?"

Offering a half-smile, she said, "A little girl from Waldorf, Maryland invited her biological mother and grandparents to dine with her this Friday. Are you free?"

Rosie jumped up and screamed, "Your baby found you?"

Jenna nodded. "Her name's Carly McCoy. Her parents are Frank and Kim McCoy." Jenna's eyes watered. "She wants me to hug her, Mom."

"Oh, honey," Rosie said, palming her chest. "I prayed so many years for this day to come." She looked at her husband. "Now we'll finally be able to know she's okay, Dom."

Dom's eyes rose above the rims of his glasses. Eyeing Jenna with less enthusiasm, he asked, "How'd she find you?"

"The family saw my picture on the front page of their local newspaper. The McCoys recognized my name."

"Why is it they know your name, but you didn't know theirs?" he asked, as if Jenna kept the details a secret from him.

Annoyed by his accusatory tone, she stood and grabbed a bottle of water from the refrigerator. "I don't know, Dad. Maybe they heard the nuns talking about me." Shooting her father a hostile stare, she asked, "Why do I feel like I'm on a witness stand, and you don't believe a word I'm saying?"

Dom rolled his eyes. "Maybe if you'd trust us, we wouldn't find ourselves in predicaments like traveling to Waldorf, Maryland to meet our granddaughter." Playing with a spoon, he escalated the tension by asking, "Is the father invited to this dinner?"

Rosie shot her husband a stare to silence him.

Dom stared back and told her, "I won't apologize because my sadness over losing my grandchild upsets you."

Rosie countered, "You're not the only one who's sad. Would you rather die never knowing her?"

Sighing, he asked, "What do any of us know about these people? What if it's a scam?"

Jenna blinked back tears. "You're right, Dad. The McCoys searched the globe and targeted your gullible daughter."

Steve's forehead creased at the rancor Jenna directed at her father. "Come on you two; we're on the same team."

Targeting Steve like a missile, Jenna shot back, "Remember that advice when your mother dredges up every mistake you've ever made since you were a toddler." Her bitterness boiled over when she turned her eyes to her father sitting at the table and said, "No matter how many times and how many ways I say I'm sorry, you still won't forgive me." Her voice shook, "All because I was a stupid kid who let myself believe I was special enough for the most popular guy on campus to love me." Choking back tears, she glared at Steve. "So, spare me the lectures. I've tried to be a good, positive person, but I'm tired of putting a filter on my disappointments." She turned to her father and yelled, "Ronan King, Dad! That's the guy who walked out on your ditzy daughter." Hot tears trickled down her cheeks as she finally purged the deep-seated anger she harbored for over a decade. "Don't worry, Dad. I can't forget what I did was wrong. You and the great *I Am* won't let me forget. God designed a punishment for me that will even the score for eternity. I'll get to know my baby in a nick of time to watch her die."

Shocked by her behavior, Steve grabbed hold of her shoulders, and said, "You're being unreasonable."

"She's dying?" Rosie whispered in shock.

Jenna wiped her eyes and said with sarcasm, "Yeah, Mom. How many candles do we light this time?"

Steve pulled a chair out for Jenna. His eyes moved from Jenna to Dom. "You two can keep fighting to be right, or we can work together to make this right."

Dom rubbed his furrowed brow with one hand as his sympathetic eyes weighed heavily on his daughter. "God's not out to get us, Jenna. Misfortune is a part of life. Tragedy's when we lose hope and give up."

More like a plea, she cried, "I can't keep the water out of the ship anymore, Daddy."

Dom stood and pulled his daughter into his arms. "Then we'll keep it out for you." He looked at his wife. "You're right. We prayed; God answered. If you two believe the McCoys are legitimate, let's sit down to supper and meet our granddaughter."

Rosie talked with Jenna on the patio while Steve and Dom discussed flight plans. An hour later, Jenna tugged gently at Steve's earlobe and said, "I have school tomorrow."

Before Steve opened the door to leave, Dom wrapped his arms around Jenna and squeezed.

She turned to him and said, "I don't want to feel guilty anymore, Dad."

He planted a soft kiss on her forehead. "We're all tired of feeling guilty, princess. Here and now, let's bury it." He held her tighter and said, "Losing your brother, losing the baby, and feeling like we lost you . . . I couldn't stop my family from slipping away."

"I want and need your support, Daddy, but I'm thirty-three years old, and I'm still afraid to make a mistake around you guys."

Dom shook his head. "Each one of us stands on a mountain of mistakes." He palmed his heart. "Some of us are fortunate to share our lives with people who forgive."

Steve reached for Jenna's hand and asked, "Would it make everyone feel better if Phil runs a background check on the McCoys? We'll know who we're dealing with by Tuesday."

Rosie said, "It wouldn't hurt."

Jenna eyed her father.

Dom drew his daughter back into his arms, swung his eyes to Steve, and said, "*Questa ragazza è il mio battito cardiaco.*"

Steve nodded saying, "I've come to treasure the heartbeat you hold in your hands."

The drive from Dulles Airport to Waldorf, Maryland seemed endless, wrought with angst mixed with excitement. The report Phil gathered confirmed the impeccable reputation of the McCoy family, leaving only one major concern. Would Carly be bedridden, having one of her bad days?

The houses in the development were inviting. Fresh sprouts of early spring green lawn stretched for blocks without a single fence posturing to keep neighbors in or out. The road began to wind uphill as Steve navigated the twists and turns drawing them closer to their destination. When they turned into the McCoy driveway, they gave each other silent looks of expectation. Dom turned to Jenna and said, "No matter what happens here today, princess, you're one brave lady."

She reached over, palmed his cheek, and said, "It's heredity, Dad."

Jenna rang the doorbell, stepped back, and raised her eyebrows in anticipation. Within seconds, Frank swung the door open and greeted them.

After the introductions, he said, "Kim's upstairs helping Carly pick out something to wear. The girl's on her twenty-seventh outfit." He guided them to the living room and poured drinks. Handing Jenna a glass of ginger ale, he said, "She's aiming to impress you."

Jenna let out a laugh, pointed to her parents, and said, "I'm still trying to impress them."

"That's hard to believe. According to that newspaper account of the school crisis, it seems you impressed the whole country."

"Those boys are the real heroes."

Turning to Steve, Frank said, "Thank you for setting this meeting up for us."

"My pleasure."

Frank's eyes blurred for only a second before he regained composure, locked eyes with Jenna, and said, "We gambled contacting you." Shaking his head, he added, "Your immediate, positive reaction surprised us. Sister Martine was adamant when she told us your desire was to walk away and never look back."

Jenna's eyes watered. "A know-it-all kid issued those instructions a lifetime ago." Her eyes briefly rested on her father before swinging back to Frank. She pulled out a tissue and dabbed her nose. "Not a day dawns and sets that I don't carry my baby in my head and heart." She looked down and dabbed the corner of her eyes. "I'm sorry for the pain I caused you, caused Carly, caused my parents."

Overcome with emotion, Jenna excused herself and wandered to the foyer to compose herself. Standing at the foot of the stairs, she overheard whispering in the upstairs hallway.

"Get moving, Carly. They came a long way to be with you, and I'm sure they're hungry."

Despite voices and laughter from the living room filtering through the house, the quiet at the top of the stairs thickened. Jenna sucked in her breath and held it for several seconds waiting to hear her daughter's voice again.

"What if she thinks I'm ugly? Look at me, Mom. I'm a skin and bones, bald freak."

Jenna's heart melted. Holding onto the staircase post, she softly called up the stairs, "What if *you* think *I'm* freaky?"

Carly peeked around the corner. Her big, brown eyes caught Jenna standing on the bottom step staring up at her. She smiled sheepishly, walked with Kim to the top step, and sat. Placing one hand on her hairless head, she said, "I used to have pretty hair like yours." She twirled a curly haired wig on the index finger of her other hand and said with dejection, "Like this stupid thing makes me look better." Keeping her eyes fixed on Jenna, she added, "I knew you'd be pretty."

Jenna climbed the stairs, knelt on the step before Carly, and said, "You're prettier." Cupping Carly's face, she planted a soft kiss on her bare head. "Anyone can be attractive with hair. Only extra-ordinary people can be as beautiful as you without hair." She enveloped Carly, and pulled her close to her heart. Holding her tightly, she whispered, "I never stopped loving you for a moment." Her eyes swung to Kim standing behind Carly. "I'm so thankful you loved her more than . . ." She caressed Carly's cheek and fought back tears.

Kim squeezed next to Carly and draped her arms around Jenna and her daughter. The three of them huddled together and cried.

Frank told the Rossis, "Excuse me for a moment while I round up the women folk." Standing at the bottom of the stairs, he shook off an impulse to join the tearful trio and suggested, "Come down and meet your grandparents."

Carly adjusted her wig on her head and made her way down the stairs behind Jenna. When she entered the living room, Dom jumped up. Unable to contain his excitement, he said, "My God, Rosie, she's the spitting image of my mother!" He extended his hand, but Carly pushed past it and flew into his arms. Looking up at him with mischief twinkling in her eyes, she yanked off her wig and asked, "Was she bald, too?"

Laughter rose from the group at the same time they marveled at Carly's casual wit in the face of terminal illness.

Rosie explained, "Not at all, sweetheart. Dom's mother had the largest darkest eyes and most beautiful skin of anyone on earth. She carried herself like royalty."

"She's my great-grandmother, right?" Carly asked.

Rosie nodded.

Carly slipped out of Dom's arms and faced Rosie. "You're the only grandmother I have now. Grandma Marty died a few months before I started to get sick."

Rosie caressed Carly's cheek then gently wrapped her arms around her grand-daughter's frail body. She closed her eyes and savored the moment.

"I want to hold you forever," Rosie whispered. "This moment is more wonderful than all of my dreams."

Carly smiled and whispered back, "I called Grandma Marty every Sunday. Can I call you?"

"Rosie planted a kiss on her cheek. "I'd be honored to share my Sundays with you, sweetheart."

Carly pointed to her father and teased, "My great-grandmother was like royalty. Maybe that's why you call me princess."

Jenna's hands flew to her mouth. "Oh my gosh!" Pointing to Dom, she said, "He calls me princess all the time."

Attempting humor of his own, Steve exaggerated his hands over his mouth and said, "Oh my gosh! Notice how they both say, 'Oh my gosh?'"

They all laughed as Jenna pointed at Steve and said, "He caught that similarity the first time we spoke on the phone last week."

"I don't know about you guys, but I'm starving," Frank announced.

He looked at Kim and asked, "Do you need any help, hon?"

She waved them into the dining room, and said, "We're all set."

Trading highlights of their lives until it neared early evening, Kim smiled at Carly, and asked, "How you holding up, honey?"

Fighting to stay alert, she begged, "Just a little longer, Mom. Puhleeze?"

Kim eyed Frank. He turned to Carly. "You know what happens when you get tired?"

Neatly folding her napkin and placing it to the side of her plate, Jenna said, "Even though she's a beautiful, young lady, I'd love to . . ." She swung her hopeful eyes to Carly. "I dreamed of tucking you in a million times."

A smile lit up Carly's face as she slipped out of her chair, grabbed Jenna's hand, and said, "Come on. I'll show you my room."

Steve said, "I'll grab the Christmas tree and carry it up the stairs. You two organize it any way you want."

Jenna steadied Carly as they climbed the stairs. They planted the tree in a corner of Carly's bedroom and decorated it with the ornaments that carried Jenna's dreams for her daughter. After they added the perfect touch, a crystal angel topper Jenna's grandmother gave her the year she passed away, Jenna cradled Carly in her arms and sang, *What Child Is This*. Carly looked up and begged for more stories chronicling Jenna's life growing up with her brother Josh. Jenna was equally enthralled listening to her daughter's animated teen-talk about friends, family, and school.

"Remember this?" Carly asked, pulling on a chain around her neck that revealed a half broken cross. "Mom and Dad gave it to me on First Holy Communion Day."

"Oh my gosh!" She lifted her half of the cross out from under her blouse and explained, "My grandmother, the one my mother and father said you resemble, gave your half to me when she came back from Italy. It was the only way I could think of to keep you close to us." Swearing Carly to silence, Jenna put her finger on her lips and whispered, "I told my mom I lost it." Running her fingers over the cross, she said, "Grandma Rossi told me it was a sign that she'd always be with me, and I wanted you to know I'd always be with you."

Carly matched the two halves of the cross and kissed it. Jenna bent her head down and kissed the cross right after her. A look of satisfaction claimed Carly's face as she quickly twisted around and laid her head in Jenna's lap. Looking up, her large inquisitive eyes studied Jenna's face for several moments.

Jenna smiled down at her and said, "Go ahead, ask."

"I don't want to get you mad or make you feel bad."

Knowing they could be on the verge of painful revelations, Jenna said, "You deserve answers."

Carly's eyes brightened. "So, what's my father like?"

Jenna stiffened.

Carly sat up and said, "Honest! You don't have to talk about him if it makes you feel bad."

Jenna shook her head. "No, baby. I just wish the story had a fairy tale ending. I wish we all could've lived happily ever after."

Carly stared at Jenna and said, "Mom always says no matter how bad life seems, if we trust God, the ending will be good."

"Your mom's right, but sometimes guilt weighs people down when they know they should've made better decisions."

"So, was he a jerk?" she asked with youthful enthusiasm.

Carly's light-hearted, low expectations of her father made it easier for Jenna to be truthful and even kinder to Ronan King than she intended.

"Your father was the handsomest guy on campus. He played around like most young boys in college. Only problem was he just didn't know how to grow up." Jenna exaggerated a swoon when she said, "I would have done anything for him." Playing with Carly's earlobe, she paused for several moments, and said, "I guess I did."

Like two sorority sisters comparing notes after an exciting date, Carly asked, "So, he talked you into sex?"

Jenna lowered her eyes and picked at the bedspread for several seconds. She looked up, pulled Carly into her arms, and said, "I really loved your father, but I learned that love is a lot more than sex. When he didn't love me back, it made me afraid to trust myself, to trust other men. I never wanted to feel that kind of pain again."

Carly pulled away in surprise. "Gosh! Aren't you glad you changed your mind? Steve's a hunk if I ever saw one."

Jenna let out a laugh. "He sure is a good-looking guy, but more importantly, he's a good man, and I love him for all the right reasons. For a lot of years, I was stuck in a daydream wondering what it would've been like to love you and your father, to be a family." Tears welled. "Sometimes I'd pretend you and your father were away on a long trip, but reality has a way of catching up with us. It hurt so much knowing I'd never have you and him in my life."

"That's not true," Carly exclaimed with youthful confidence. Shrugging, she added, "So, he's a jerk, and you'll never have him in your life, but half your dream came true. You have me in your life." Her bald head made her eyes look even larger as they bulged with assurance.

"I remember when Paul Moody stopped dancing with me at our eighth-grade dance. He shoved me aside and chased after the prettiest girl in the class."

Jenna squinted in mock puzzlement. "Was Paul Moody blind? He already was dancing with the prettiest girl in the class."

"Yeah, right," she said with a shrug. She told Jenna, "I walked up to him and pushed him out of the way, and he fell on his rear." She covered her mouth with her hands and giggled as if it happened that very second. "I didn't mean to shove him that hard," she said, her eyes pleading innocence, "but he made me so mad."

Jenna hi-fived her. "That's my girl!"

"The next week, Paul jogged over here and handed me an invitation to his birthday party."

"Oh my gosh! Did you go?"

"I tore up the invitation, threw it in his face, and told him to invite Shannon Cooper." With an air of defiance, she said, "Mom wanted me to give him another chance, but I said I don't ever wanna be second best." Proud of herself, she quipped, "I take after you."

Jenna let out a laugh. "There does tend to be a hint of arrogance about us."

Carly shrugged. "My father hurt you; so why should you go back? You found someone better." She lay back down and placed her head in Jenna's lap. "I bet if I had time, I'd find someone way better than Paul Moody." She looked up at Jenna, blinked several times, and asked, "Who needs a guy anyway? I'm happy right now because all the while I searched for you, I never thought I'd really get a chance to meet you. Being with you, hearing your voice, it's like I've known you forever."

"Is one day good enough?" Jenna asked with hope in her voice.

The gaunt teen wrestled with her bedspread and slipped between her sheets. Her eyes tiring, she looked up at Jenna, and said, "It's more than good enough." More serious than she had been all evening, she locked eyes with Jenna, and said, "I thought you hated me for ruining your life." She blinked back tears. "Mom kept telling me a hateful person wouldn't have visited the convent and prayed in the chapel like you used to do." Brushing her eyes dry with her pajama sleeve, she said, "You found me the best parents in the world, and you came the first time I called you."

Continuing to survey each line, each feature of Jenna's face as though she planned to memorize it and carry it through eternity, Carly told her, "Thank you for loving me." Her voice cracked, when she added, "And thank you for giving me a chance to say, 'I love you' back."

Jenna sat on the edge of the bed and lay across Carly's frail body. She gently brushed her cheek back and forth on Carly's bare head. "Next time, we'll start the visit early in the morning so we can have all day to talk and laugh and maybe even do some shopping, okay? We'll talk until the sun peeks over the mountains." Pulling a light sheet to Carly's chin, she said, "In the meantime, you can call me anytime, day or night. I'll stop whatever I'm doing to be with you."

Carly's fingers whimsically played with Jenna's curls. Her voice sounded weaker. "I've been having more and more bad days, Jenna. It was a miracle we found you, and you came as soon as I called. It won't be long before I—"

Jenna sat up, grabbed Carly's shoulders, and said, "No! Don't talk like that."

Carly smiled knowingly. With a surge of strength, she said, "It's true. The only reason why I fought so hard was because I needed to find you." She closed her eyes for several seconds before saying, "Now I can rest."

"Do you expect me to walk out that door knowing I'll never see you again?"

"You did it once before," Carly told her innocently. "This time it will be easier."

Jenna shook her head. "Letting you go wasn't easy the first time, and it's even harder now."

"It will be," Carly said convincingly. "This time you'll know who I am. You'll know where I am, and you'll know I'm happy. I know you love me, and you know I love you." Her eyelids weighed heavily as she struggled to stay awake. Her voice was barely audible when she mumbled, "Heaven's a place where we'll all be together again. I know he'll love us in heaven." Opening her eyes for a moment, she said, "My father can't be all bad if you loved him."

Jenna caressed Carly's forehead. She held her baby's hand to her lips and kissed each finger. Sitting still at the edge of Carly's bed, she closed her eyes and lost herself in a lifetime of hopes and dreams she shared with her child in a single day that she didn't want to end. Gregorian chants echoed in the corridors of her mind when Kim's quiet knock on the door propelled her back to the stark reality that lay before her. Unable to draw herself away from the treasure her heart longed to hold, she dabbed her eyes and pleaded, "Just a little longer?"

Kim nodded.

Jenna gently placed her lips on Carly's ear and whispered, "I never felt more complete than in this moment, holding you next to my heart." She planted a soft kiss on her dying child's cheek and quietly slipped out the door.

Four weeks later, a week before commencement, the Rossis mingled with other mourners in the McCoy backyard. The white blossoms of the snow crabapple trees swayed softly in the fragrant breeze as Kim motioned for Jenna and Rosie to sit with her under a swaying shade tree. Stealing a moment to catch her breath after the emotional funeral service, she handed Jenna a wooden box tied with a gold bow.

"Carly was adamant about you having this." She hugged Jenna and said, "Every item in this box mattered to her."

Rosie, dabbing her eyes with a tissue, sat close to Jenna as Jenna lifted the lid and gently separated the orchid tissue that preserved the broken crucifix she gave her baby the day she placed her in Sister Martine's arms. Her hands shook as she ran her finger over each jagged edge of the cross. She unfolded the note she remembered writing to the nameless, faceless woman who she hoped would hold her little girl to her heart. The long ago lost and alone feeling washed over her. Careful not to tear the yellowed paper weakened at the creases by time, she folded it and placed it on her lap.

Another note carrying the fresh scent of brown sugar and figs read:

Dear Mom,

I hope you marry Steve and have a baby that you can hold in your arms and love every day. Give my half of the cross to the baby. Great-grandma and I want you to decorate the tree and tell the baby all the family stories you told me, and tell my brother or sister we're watching over all of you with love. I gathered these stone hearts from every beach we visited over the years because they reminded me of you. I hope they remind you how much I want you to live happily ever after.

Thank you for loving me first.

Carly

Included in the box was a flash drive. A note attached read,

"P.S.

Send this recording to my father. I love him, even though he didn't have a chance to love me."

Jenna's eyes blurred as she laid her head upon Rosie's shoulder, and asked, "How'd you find the strength to move through life with so much joy after losing Josh?"

Rosie raised Jenna's hand to her lips. "Josh and Carly would want us to forget them altogether rather than have their memories cause us sadness. That's reason enough to make our hearts a forgiving and joyful place for their spirits to rest."

Chapter Sixteen

Only two weeks since Carly's funeral and off the heels of a hectic graduation ceremony, Jenna was appreciative her parents talked her into a getaway on the Florida coast. The sun hung low in the early evening sky as she plodded along the shoreline. Waves crashing against distant crags and the haunting sound of seagulls magnified the desolation weighing on her heart. How was anyone supposed to fill a lifetime of love into a few sporadic days, she thought. On those days, she prayed the sun would never set.

The phone jarred her out of thought.

"Hope I'm not interrupting you," Steve told her.

"Hardly," she said, devoid of feeling. "I'm like a patch of seaweed caught in a sand puddle."

"There's no way getting around the heartache, Jen, but we'll get through this together. Things here are squared away. After landing this morning, I helped Mike get his summer schedule, and I met his roommates and some parents. We took the boys out to eat and dropped them off at the dorm. I'm catching a flight out tonight to spend some time with you."

Her uncharacteristic quietness worried him until she said, "The only way I'll be okay is if I tie up some loose ends."

"What's that supposed to mean?"

As if she didn't hear him, she recited a litany of regrets: "I wish I would've never met Ronan King. I wish I would've let my mother and father help me raise my baby. I wish I never would've known Carly was sick. I wish she didn't have to die when mean-spirited people all over this earth get to live and spread hate while all she did was love. I wish I would've told Ronan about the baby and—"

"Jesus, Jen, you're wishing for a new life. Don't do this to yourself. Don't do this to us." With a heavy sigh, he said, "All things considered, Carly was a happy kid. Both your dreams came true."

"My dream was to be her mother and—"

"And what? Be Ronan's wife?"

"I never gave him a chance to do the right thing."

"How do you expect him to do the right thing now?"

Disregarding his objections, she said, "Carly wanted him to have this recording, so I'm going to give him the recording. I'll call you when I get back."

"Why not mail him the flash drive?"

Her voice was insistent. "I need to find out how he would've—"

"Admit it, Jenna. This isn't about Carly's recording. You still need Ronan King's attention."

Although surprised by his uncharacteristic anger, she offered little consolation to alleviate his hurt feelings when she countered, "I'm sorry you don't understand, but I'm tired of explaining myself."

Letting his jealousy get the best of him, he upbraided her. "You're not the only one who's tired. I'm tired of trying to compete with your fantasies of Ronan holding you in his arms and mourning with you. Isn't it enough that Carly loved you? That I love—"

"You have no right to tell me how I should feel or act or what should be sufficient to heal my sadness."

Pausing for a second, he countered, "Loving you gives me the right to tell you how I feel and how I want you to act. How you respond reflects how much I mean to you." After a short silence between them, he said with exasperation, "Do what you want, but don't expect me to wait around to make love to you while all you're thinking about is Ronan King."

"This isn't about loving Ronan. I need to know—"

Provoked by what he perceived as a selfish pursuit, Steve told her, "Mark this down on your need to know list. You need to know that I need to know if your heart is still with me."

Anxious to exit the noisy airport terminal, she hailed a cab from JFK to the Hyatt. She freshened up in her room before sitting at the bar to order a ginger ale loaded with ice. Unintentionally sounding like a reporter, she told the bartender, "My favorite professor told us, 'If you want to know the buzz, get to know the secretaries, janitors, and bartenders.'"

Wiping the bar in front of her, the burly man with thick, black framed glasses laughed, and asked, "So, what's the lady wanna know?"

She swirled her drink and asked, "Do you know a painless way to contact a politician running for office?"

"All politicians are pains in the ass, but it helps if I have a name," he teased, collecting ice into a bucket.

"Ronan King."

The bartender's big, round eyes rolled. "Give the alley cat a few minutes and his radar'll pick up the scent of a pretty lady like you," he said, snapping his fingers, "like that."

Sipping her drink to calm the knot in her stomach, she asked, "That bad?"

A business man sitting to her right overheard the conversation. Downing the last portion of his whiskey, he turned to Jenna, and quipped, "King would have to evolve another thousand years just to reach slime status."

Her heart drooped.

Forcing a matter-of-fact tone, she asked, "A womanizer, huh?"

The bartender slid another whiskey highball on the rocks to the business man, shrugged, and said, "That's puttin' it gently."

"With such a vile reputation, what makes him believe he's going to win the race?"

Wiping his hands with the bar rag, the bartender eyed her, and said, "Money and softball-size nads—excuse my language—are pretty persuasive allies."

The businessman agreed saying, "And this King guy has a helluva lot of both."

The bartender shrugged again. "If people throw golf balls at the wall of life, a golf ball's gonna come bouncin' back at them. Ronan King tosses garbage at the wall of life, and if people elect him, they better not be surprised when a whole lot of waste starts flyin' around this city."

"Now that I know what to expect, how do I contact Mr. King?"

"King's campaign headquarters is ten blocks away. Any cab driver will reluctantly get you there." The bartender leaned closer to Jenna and whispered, "Cabbies hate his guts. He's messin' with their livelihood."

Slipping off her barstool, she asked, facetiously, "Do I need to hire a bodyguard?"

With raised eyebrows, the bartender pointed at her, and warned, "Just don't fall for his phony crap. Underneath all the glitz and glamour slithers and slides a cobra."

At the King headquarters, the secretary raised her eyes over the rims of her glasses and stared at Jenna standing on the other side of the desk.

"May I help you?"

"I need to discuss an important matter with Ronan—"

The secretary stood, picked up a folder, and walked toward the file cabinet. "What you need is an appointment." She grabbed several papers from the fax machine and stuffed them in another already burgeoning folder. Walking back to her desk, she said with detachment, "He won't be back until five; he has a dinner date at six, and he's booked for the rest of the week."

Tired of languishing in doubt and carrying the fresh wounds of losing Carly, the secretary's attitude stirred a heated response from Jenna. She stepped in the woman's path, and said, "Tell Ronan King he'll lose this election tonight if he doesn't give me ten minutes of his time."

Jenna's eyes dared the woman to defy her.

The secretary pulled back and eyed Jenna with angry suspicion. More to get rid of her than comply with her threat, she asked Jenna, "Where can he reach you?"

"I'm staying at the Hyatt." Jenna bent down, picked scrap paper off the floor, and scrawled her name and number on the back of the paper. "He may recognize the name. I expect to talk with him before this night's over."

Waiting in her room for Ronan's call grated on her nerves. She dozed off reading a local paper when the phone startled her to attention. His voice was soft and seductive.

"Jenna Rossi, please."

"Hello, Ronan. It's been a long time."

"Jenna," he whispered in a throaty voice. "To what do I owe this pleasure?"

Picturing him in a velvet smoking jacket, pouring a glass of Cabernet Sauvignon, she said, "We need to talk."

After a short coughing spell, he apologized saying, "You handled that hostage situation like a Navy Seal."

The thought of Carly drifting off saying, "If you loved him, he can't be all bad," calmed her.

"I require nothing from you except time to give you a recording from a mutual friend and tell you something I should've told you fourteen years ago. Meet me at the Hyatt at five. I'll be sure you make your six o'clock dinner date."

"Forget dinner. I'd rather recapture the magic."

Swallowing hard, she said, "I'm not peddling magic, Ronan. What I have to say is real."

She hung up, took a deep breath, and whispered facetiously, "Magic?" A shiver ran through her body. Talking aloud to no one there, she said, "He emptied himself into me like an animal in heat. He walks away while I have his baby in a foreign country, and now he wants to capture the magic." Rankled by his arrogance, she grabbed a pillow and punched it hard. All I want to know is if Carly would've made a difference to you, she thought.

The moment she entered the hotel dining room, the hostess whisked her off to the secluded VIP section. Ronan stood and sensually perused her from head to foot.

"You're more beautiful today than the day I made love to you."

Put off by his forward demeanor, Jenna waited for the waitress to fill their glasses with water and promise to return to take their orders before she asked, "Are you sure you made love, Ronan? Rumor has it you delight in screwing women."

Letting out a fraudulent laugh, he said, "Leave it to an English teacher to complicate the issue with semantics."

"The inability to distinguish the difference between the two concepts is what complicates life." Wiping the condensation from her glass, she said, "I'll get to the point."

Offering Jenna wine he had ordered before she arrived, he coughed some more, and asked as though he were conspiring with her, "Why are we even in this crowded place?" His smile crinkled his eyes as he canvassed her face. Wiping his fingers on a napkin, he said, "Let's get a room, relax, and talk about what we both want."

Jenna declined the wine and scanned the busy hotel restaurant buzzing with heightened activity. A guest at the hotel or maybe an excited diner had notified the media that Ronan King was dining in the hotel restaurant, making him an easy target for media. As the hotel manager held the reporters at bay, Jenna's phone rang.

"I need to take this call. It's a close friend experiencing a rough patch in her life."

Relieved to sit back and absorb the beauty of her presence in his life once more, Ronan nodded and listened to Jenna calm Samantha Kind.

"Thank God you answered, Jen!" Her voice fell into an infantile whine. "Flashbacks are so scary. It's really hard. My mom let him hurt me. Why? Why didn't they love me, Jen? My analyst said I need people to hold me. I want people to hold me; I really do, but every time a guy tries to hold me, I gag. Sometimes I even throw up. Thank God, my analyst holds me. Sometimes I'm even afraid to keep my appointments. I never gagged when Josh put his arm around me. I miss little Josh so much. Why does God make the wrong people die? Your mom used to hug me and call me an angel. That's why she always made me angel hair pasta."

When Sam paused to take a breath, Jenna told her, "I can't talk right now. I'm sitting in a New York restaurant taking care of important business."

"Why'd you answer the phone if you can't talk?" Resentment swelled, causing her to lash out. "Go ahead; take care of business while my life's falling apart. I'm getting drunk as hell, and I plan to stay drunk." After several loud sniffles, more child-like, she pleaded, "I don't mean it, Jen. Honest." Whispering, she told Jenna, "I'm just so scared. I'm stuck. Half the time I can't tell if I'm living back when I was eight, or right now. Life's one gigantic blur. I'm thirty-three, but I feel like a three-year-old, and I'm always so scared."

The sound of liquid pouring into a glass clinking against the phone unnerved Jenna. Sam continued to nag saying, "You're always telling me how you can't come here because you live an hour away, but by golly, you found time to board a plane to take care of business with God knows who you're with." After a gulp of whiskey, she asked, "So, who's more important than me this time, Jenna?" Before Jenna could explain, Sam said, "Never mind; who cares anyway?"

"Sam?"

The silence weighed heavy on her already burdened heart.

Jenna slipped the phone into her purse, looked at Ronan, and said, "Sorry for the interruption."

Letting out a sarcastic laugh, he asked, "Is that the same friend who always bugged you in college?" Eyeing her with a mix of confusion and admiration, he asked, "What makes you care about someone so hopeless after all these years?"

"My dad gave me the world. Sam's father held the key to his Ford Ranger over a fire and literally branded her right shoulder. Besides," she said flippantly, "sometimes sharing the burdens of frail friends is easier than pacifying ingrates who abuse the blessings they've been given."

Externally keeping his emotional distance, he sat in the silence she gave him to retreat. He had never forgotten her unvarnished honesty, and occasionally longed for what he let slip away that night long ago. In his world where love was nonexistent, she remained a distant star flickering in his bleak universe. He reminded himself how he came close to destroying every good thing about her.

Clutching the flash drive Carly wanted her to give him, Jenna said, "I'm here to come clean. I withheld vital information from you all these years. What you do with the knowledge now is up to you."

"You have my attention."

Emptying herself of fear, she said, "Let's get back to semantics for a moment. I made love to you; you screwed me."

Shaking his head in opposition to mask his hurt at her inability to appreciate the unique place she held in his heart, he leaned across the table, and said, "No, Jenna. You underestimate the favor I did you when I rushed you out of my frat house."

Fighting the urge to retreat, she fixed her eyes on him and countered, "No doubt, but I did you a bigger favor. I gave birth to a baby girl." She slid the flash drive across the table, kept her fingers on it, and said, "She wanted you to have this because—"

Ronan's jaw stiffened. His face reddened as he commanded through clenched teeth, "Stop right there!" A hard cough interrupted his impending verbal attack. He gathered phlegm in a napkin and wrapped it in a tight ball. Eyes blazing, a familiar bullying disposition seized him. Pointing at her, he said, "Say one more word, and if she proves mine, I'll sue for custody and make sure you never lay eyes on her again." Without blinking, he reached for a clean napkin, wiped his brow, and slammed it on the table. Confused by her apparent commonality with the other women in his life, he said with a sneer, "I suggest you get up right now, waltz out that door, and pray I forget this conversation ever took place."

Despite the heat from his hot, piercing stare, an inexplicable calm moved Jenna to say, "I'm prepared to waltz out that door and answer a few questions from that pool of eager reporters, then forget you altogether." Playing with the edge of her napkin, she said, "Your inability to appreciate your part in creating a precious little girl whose heart was devoid of bitterness toward either of us for giving her up is stunning." Jenna's eyes fell when she admitted, "But it's my fault you didn't know she was alive all these years." Twisting her napkin tighter, she leveled a cold indictment. "Your reaction today is even more detestable than I imagined it would have been fourteen years ago." With a sadder voice, she said, "For years, I resisted believing the vile rumors that dogged you." Fighting the mist clouding her eyes, she told him, "But I can't excuse your cold, callous reaction today toward our innocent child who died loving us. I can and will hold that against you."

She flung her dirty napkin toward him and stood to leave. He jumped up, grabbed her arm, and asked with unmistakable relief in his voice, "The girl's dead?"

She turned and scanned him from sole to crown. His traitor eyes gave her the impetus to say, "I anticipated cold and selfish, but pernicious joy of a child's death?" She shook her head with disdain. "Your beautiful daughter's name was Carly, and yes, she's dead. I don't know what she said to you, but also dead is the iota of good she or anyone else will ever truthfully attribute to your miserable existence."

Breathing more steadily, he sat back down. Angry with himself for miscalculating her intent, he softened telling her, "I over-reacted. Let me make it up to you." Trying to delay her departure, he foolishly proposed, "Let's start over."

Crossing her arms over her chest, she faked a shiver. "I'm not in to emotionally and spiritually challenged men." Sad and tired, she said, "Your purpose is to serve New York on your own."

"It's encouraging to know you believe I have a purpose."

Jutting her jaw, she said, "We all have a purpose in life, Ronan. A moral eunuch like you will make a perfect asshole for New York."

His heart sank. Confusion filled his once arrogant eyes as he watched her swagger toward the lobby. A swarm of reporters aimed microphones toward her face.

"What's your connection to Ronan King?"

Fighting to subdue the adrenalin rush her release from Ronan King afforded her only moments before, she said, "We have a mutual friend."

Another reporter asked, "Do you plan to support Ronan King in his bid for election?"

"My mission was merely to fulfill a promise to our mutual friend."

"Will you play a role in his campaign?" the reporter badgered.

"No. I expect New Yorkers will vote for candidates who demonstrate depth of feeling and a sincere capacity to extend themselves beyond selfish wants and needs."

"Are you calling Ronan King shallow and selfish?"

Jenna smiled at the persistent reporter, and said, "If voters want a just and caring community, they should avoid voting for self-centered, narcissistic con men."

The burly hotel bartender watching the television screen on the wall above the bar ran his hand through his curly hair and said to one of his customers, "How 'bout that!" Pointing to the screen, he said, "I warned that lady about Ronan King a few hours ago." He punched his fist in the air. "She nailed him."

Ronan King sat dazed, pondering what had transpired. Jenna had no way of knowing that her revelation and unique refusal to ask anything of him stirred an unusual longing for her. The ring tone on his phone diverted his attention to weightier matters.

"Ronan? Doctor Young. We need to talk."

"How bad is it?"

"I'm afraid there are no good options."

Ronan slipped Carly's flash drive into his blazer pocket and walked away.

Chapter Seventeen

JENNA PHONED HER MOTHER AND SAID, "I'M HOME."

"Oh, Jenna, we were so worried about you. We're flying home tomorrow afternoon. Did you get in touch with Steve?"

Holding the phone in the crook of her neck as she unpacked, she asked, "What's the use? He practically gave me an ultimatum before I flew to New York."

"Can you blame him? We're all trying to understand why you ran off. When you get an idea in your head, you—"

"Stop, Mom." Tired and seething from Ronan's despicable attitude toward Carly's death, she snobbishly countered, "Don't nag me."

Shifting the conversation to avoid a confrontation, Rosie asked, "So, what did this Ronan have to say?"

"He's self-centered and cold, but I'm finally free of him. Telling him I was pregnant back then would've made it worse for everyone concerned." Pausing, she said, "The only regret I can't shake is not telling you. Carly would've been ours."

"Jenna, the McCoys shared her with us because Carly was always ours."

A quiet moment passed before Jenna sighed and said, "For the first time in years, I feel like I can finally be myself, open and honest about my life."

"Baby, don't forget that Steve loves you."

"I hope he does," she said, her voice soft with regret. "I'll call him tomorrow and thank him for being my best friend throughout this ordeal."

"Come on, Jenna." Rosie gently chastised. "He's more than a friend."

Irritated by Rosie's insistence, she asked, "You want me to grovel?"

"I want you to—"

"Not this time, Mom. I'd rather be road-kill for maggots before I beg another man to love me."

Rosie rolled her eyes. "Maybe some sleep will curb that exaggeration."

The incessant ringing of the doorbell woke Jenna from a deep sleep. Tripping two times on her way to the door, she yawned wide, and said, "Come in, Lizzy, before you wake up the whole apartment complex."

"It's ten o'clock in the morning, Sleeping Beauty. The rest of the world's been hustling and bustling for hours."

"Things at rest tend to stay at rest," Jenna said through another yawn.

Fumbling the yellow Lab puppy she was carrying, Lizzy said, "I need a dog sitter for this mutt Jerry dropped in my lap while you were away." The puppy squirmed out of Lizzy's arms and slipped to the floor with a soft thud. Disoriented at first, the dog yelped, ran in circles, then scampered to Jenna's feet and began licking her toes.

Jenna bent down and sang, "Look at you, little peanut." She lifted the pup and cradled it in her arms. The puppy immediately scooted into the crook between Jenna's neck and ear where it nibbled her earlobe.

"That's gratitude for yah," Lizzy exclaimed. "She whines and growls at me like a she-wolf and laps you up like you're a hot-fudge sundae sprinkled with puppy chow."

"Chocolate's not good for puppies. Maybe this little peanut senses you don't want her," Jenna countered, cooing at the puppy as she talked.

"Then the mutt's perceptive," Lizzy said with a mirthful tone.

Jenna held the puppy up to her face and planted a soft kiss between its eyes. The puppy reciprocated with several wet, warm licks to Jenna's nose and cheek.

"Too bad this love fest's only going to last a day because this dog has a date with the pound tomorrow."

"Come on, Lizzy," Jenna cooed to the puppy. "The last place this little peanut belongs is in a pound."

"I honestly can't take care of her, Jen. All she does is poop, cry, and poop some more." More seriously, Lizzy said, "This is the calmest that animal has been in three days. You want her; she's yours. Otherwise, address your love letters to the Humane Society."

"Does she have food and a cage, or do I have to go shopping?"

"Are you serious?" Lizzy asked with hope in her voice.

"Why not?" Jenna countered. Gently running her index finger between the puppy's eyes, she said, "It might be therapeutic to have a living thing in my life that showers me with unconditional love."

Before Jenna had a chance to change her mind, Lizzy ran next door, gathered the dog's paraphernalia, and carted it to Jenna's apartment. Leaning the last piece of the cage up against the back of Jenna's couch, she proclaimed, "Once I walk out that door, a *no return policy* automatically goes into effect."

"You're free, Lizzy. Have fun. Noce Baby and I need our rest."

Lizzy narrowed her eyes. "What kind of name is *Noce Baby*?"

Trading soft kisses with the puppy, Jenna said, "Noce rhymes with coach. It means *nut* in Italian. She's my little peanut, my Noce Baby."

"Well, your precious Noce Baby hasn't slept in a day and a half, and neither have I. Final warning: You sure you're up for this responsibility?"

Nuzzling the puppy, Jenna said, "For better or worse, 'til death do us part."

Lizzy raised her hands high over her head and shouted, "Hallelujah! Now I know how Atlas felt when some sucker came along and lifted the world off his shoulders."

"Hercules wasn't a sucker." Jenna cuddled Noce and teased, "It didn't take him long to trick Atlas into holding up the heavens again." With one brow raised, she shot Lizzy a fake, sinister look, and warned, "You better scram before I—"

Lizzie jumped up, swung open the door, and said, "I'm outta here nutty buddies. May you and Noce have a long-lasting love affair."

Jenna sprawled on the couch and let Noce wander over her body until she circled on her chest two times and gently plopped down. Several seconds later, Noce scooted up and nestled her nose between Jenna's neck and ear. She felt the puppy's warm, soft puffs of sleepy breath on her neck. The rapid beat of the puppy's heart steadied as Jenna's slow, rhythmic heart beat calmed the creature to sleep.

So, this is what Steve longs for, she thought. She gently played with the puppy's ear, and whispered, "Maybe you can teach me a trick or two, little one."

Jenna stretched to reach the phone ringing on the end-table. Noce wiggled, licked Jenna's cheek several times with her warm, wet tongue, and closed her eyes and fell back into blissful sleep.

Rosie announced, "We're back, sweetie." Sounding tired, she said, "I plan to unpack, shower, and take a cat-nap."

Jenna let out a laugh. "Funny how people go away to relax, and the first thing they do when they get home is crave sleep. I've been lounging all day."

"Any word from Steve?"

"No, Mom. Besides, I've been devoting myself to a new love in my life."

Jenna cringed at her mother's heavy sigh of disapproval.

"I honestly don't know what you want out of life, Jen. Steve is perfect for you. If you're not more considerate of his feelings, you're going to lose—"

"Lighten up, Mom. Listen."

She gently poked Noce with her index finger until the puppy let out several soft whimpers.

"Are you with some kind of animal?" her mother asked.

"It's the cutest yellow Lab puppy. Lizzy planned to drop it off at the pound, but the little peanut fell asleep on me, so I decided to adopt it and name her Noce."

Jubilation sprang from Rosie's lips. "A puppy's a wonderful idea. Remember when you and Josh used to play with Patches?"

Jenna laughed. "How about when Dad bought that gigantic television set for us. Remember how Josh and I spent hours transforming the huge box into our playhouse? Gosh," she said, her voice filled with longing. "How we waited for weekends. You'd let us camp out on the porch and sleep in the box with Patches."

Rosie's voice turned sad. "I almost forgot that. Time sure has a way of editing our memories." After a pause, she said, "Some days I struggle to remember your brother's sweet voice; I feel guilty when I forget the littlest notions about him." After a shorter pause, she said, "I miss him so much, Jen. Maybe that's why we hover over you more than we should."

"I know, Mom. I miss him, too. I'm a bigger pain than Josh ever was, but don't give up on me yet."

"I will never give up on you, baby. Just don't be too hard on Steve. He's a good man." Sighing, she said, "Right now I'm hitting the showers. Kiss that peanut for me, and tell her I'm thrilled beyond words that she's a dog."

By late afternoon Jenna was feeling miles apart from Steve. She scooped Noce up and said, "Come on, peanut; let's take a ride to the top of Sparta."

Noce lay content on the passenger seat of the jeep as Jenna drove to Steve's special spot overlooking the city. Pulling up to the dirt road leading up to the top of the hill, she jumped out and slipped a bright, red, oversized collar on the puppy and allowed her to dawdle and sniff her way to the top. Standing at the summit, Jenna's eyes surveyed the valley below. In awe of the hazy sun hanging low in the rosy-colored sky, an hour passed as she sat on a large rock paying little attention to the darker, more ominous clouds rolling in from the west.

Restless, Noce yelped and tugged on her leash until she wiggled her way out of the collar and playfully bounded toward the thicket.

Jenna jumped up and ordered her to come back. Mumbling under her breath, she looked at the sky, and asked, "Why does it have to be one storm after another?"

Dark clouds blanketed the hilltop as the dog's yelping grew faint. Unfamiliar with the terrain, she was hesitant to traipse deeper into the brush to retrieve the puppy. Scanning the edge of the thicket, she spotted a small animal's carcass picked to the bone.

Dizzying, she said to no one there, "Please don't let me lose her, too."

Seeming to mock her fear, a bolt of lightning lit up the dark sky and sent her lurching backward. Several seconds later, thunder rolled across the heavens shaking the earth below as dark clouds let loose a torrential rain.

"Noce!" she screamed.

More loud thunder rumbling through the sky swallowed up her terrified voice. She carefully shuffled through the mud, sat on the knee-high boulder, and wrapped her arms around her knees. Hard drops of rain steadily pelted her already wet body. She bent her head down to her knees and bit her bottom lip with such intensity, her teeth felt as though they'd come out the other side. Tears mixed with rain. A touch on her shoulder caused her to jump up and spin around.

"No sorrow's worth drowning a whole city."

Stunned at the sight of him, she stuttered, "I . . . I shouldn't be here. I lost my. . ." She covered her face with her hands.

Equally drenched as she was, Steve eyed her sympathetically, and said, "I'm feeling lost myself."

Wiping her face with her hands, she said, "I wanted to show my puppy how beautiful it is up here before . . ." Her eyes rolled across the terrain. Overcome with futility, she said, "I lost her like I lose everything."

He draped his arm across her shoulders and steadied her trembling body. Pulling her close, he used his flashlight to guide her back to the boulder. She sat first; he straddled her from behind.

"These flash storms pass quickly. Let's sit tight and ride it out." Several minutes of silence passed when the torrent turned into gentle drops lighting on them bound close together. The rumbling of thunder sounded distant, and dark clouds gave way to a lighter evening sky.

He placed his lips on her ear and said, "You must hold a special love for that puppy to sit up here in a nasty storm waiting for her to come back."

"I do love her, Steve. Just because she ran away, doesn't mean she wants to be somewhere else. The storm caused her to lose direction." Running her damp sleeve over her face, she said, "I'll never forgive myself if some animal drags her off."

Resting his chin on her head full of wet curls, he told her, "I never would've forgiven myself if some animal dragged you off in New York."

She turned and stared at him wide-eyed.

Locking eyes with her, he said, "Trust me, Jen. The only animal on this property big enough to carry away a Lab pup is a human being."

"How'd you know Noce was a Lab?"

Shrugging, he asked, "Any chance you could love me as enthusiastically as you love the dog resting in the cab of my truck?"

She caressed his cheek. "Despite what you and my parents think, I didn't wander away in pursuit of Ronan King. Why can't you believe that?"

Ignoring her question, he pointed upward. The early evening sky began to hug the horizon with a deep shade of purple veined with pale blue.

"Isn't that a magnificent sight?"

Jenna fixed her eyes on the beauty unfolding above her when Steve directed the flashlight to a patch of mud in front of them and asked with exaggerated excitement, "What the heck is that?"

She jumped up, looked down past her mud-caked shoes, and caught sight of the object. She gently slapped his shoulder, and said, "My gosh, Steve. I thought you saw a snake."

Laughing, he crouched to pick up the object.

Continuing to shine the light on it, he sat back on the boulder, and she curled close in front of him. Inspecting it more closely, he said, "It's just an old ring." He turned off the flashlight and laid it on the ground. Locking eyes with her, he held the ring up, and asked nonchalantly, "Keep it, or toss it?"

Holding out her hand, she said, "Let me clean it off first." She rinsed the ring in a nearby puddle, brushed it dry on her pant leg, and said, "This is no ordinary ring. Look how it shines."

"Really?" he asked, taking it from her to inspect it more closely.

Her eyes widened as he lifted her hand, slipped the ring on her finger, and said, "An extra-ordinary ring belongs on the hand of an extra-ordinary woman."

Jenna raised her hand close to her face and stared at the ring. Swinging her eyes to him, she whispered, "Is this for real?"

"As real as we make it."

Her lips grabbed his and lingered until he broke away, and asked, "Is that a yes?"

Planting a soft kiss on his lips, she whispered, "Oh, yes."

She wiped the ring clean with her wet jersey and held her hand up close to her face to admire it again. "I never saw a ring as beautiful as this."

"There's no other like it, Jenna. My grandfather designed it himself. He was so crazy in love with my grandmother; he bartered with every jeweler across Italy to get the perfect stones for it. It was his gift to her for loving him enough to leave her family behind and sail away with him to America."

"Did Amy wear it, too?" she asked, trying hard to mask the twinge of jealousy in her voice.

"Oh, no! Only my grandmother; now you. When I told my mother I was flying to Florida to be with you, to ask you to be with me for the rest of my life, she offered me the ring. When you insisted on flying to New York, it threw a cog in my plan."

"Why didn't she give it to Phil and Susan?"

"Phil didn't tell my parents he was getting engaged, and Sue's quite enamored with that cheap costume jewel Phil slipped on her finger at the State Fair."

"Phil's not cheap."

"He didn't buy the ring. They were walking on a path at the fair at dusk, and he spotted it on the ground. He picked it up, slipped it on her finger and told her, "Say you'll marry me before the sun goes down, and I'll always have sunshine in my life."

"Oh my gosh! How romantic is that?"

Steve let out a laugh. "That piece of junk makes her finger turn black, but the only way she'll remove it is if someone chops off her finger."

Jenna stared at her ring and then back at him. "I love this ring, but you know what I love more?"

"Noce?"

She tapped his wet, cold nose and said, "More than the puppy."

"What then?"

"I love that you trust me."

He tightened his arms around her and said, "These past few days, I was skeptical." Pressing his cheek to hers, he admitted, "I was relieved to see your jeep below. I figured you wouldn't be on our hill if your heart was with," he exaggerated the name, *Ronan*.

Her sympathetic eyes canvassed his face before she said, "You were so angry. I couldn't convince you that meeting Ronan had nothing to do with love." Palming his cheek, she said, "I love you, but I needed to know if not telling him about Carly was the colossal mistake I made it out to be all these years."

"Did you find your answer?"

Pushing his damp hair off his forehead, she said, "He was visibly relieved when I told him Carly was dead."

Steve winced.

"By now he's listened to Carly's recording. She probably forgave him like she forgave me. He'd have to be demonic to ignore her angelic voice echoing in his hollow head and heart." She laid her head on his chest. "Maybe someday he'll understand that Carly was the only good he ever created in his life."

Steve looked up at the sky and let out a hyperbolic sigh. "I feel like a Stradivarius being played by a perfect bow." More seriously, he said, "Your strokes draw music from places inside me I never knew existed."

Gently patting his head, she played with his words. "Place me here, and I'm a bow that makes the package look good, too."

Breaking into a wide grin, he told her, "A few strategic strokes can make the package feel good, too."

Jumping up, she tossed her wet hair back, and asked seductively, "Did Columbia teach you how to direct every conversation to your carnal desires?"

Innocently defending himself, he told her, "I can't help it if your sloppy word choice turns me on. If the *bow* is offering either to make me look good or feel good, I prefer the latter."

She pulled him up by his belt buckle, and said, "Now is not the time for a concert, cowboy. Let's check on Noce Baby and then show off my ring to four of our favorite people." She waved her hand in front of his face. "Tell me something. What kind of man carries an heirloom in his shirt pocket and drops it in a mud puddle in the middle of a thunderstorm?"

He jutted his jaw. "I drove to your house first. I had intentions of proposing if I felt confident you had Ronan King out of your system. You weren't home." He looked past her out over the city and paused for several seconds. "I assumed you were with him. I drove up here to jump off this cliff."

"Oh my gosh! We saved each other's lives," she teased.

Clasping hands, they laughed together as they slogged down the slippery dirt road.

"Rain on a wedding day symbolizes good fortune. I wonder what it means at an engagement."

Closing the door to her jeep, he leaned through the open window and pecked her on the cheek. Giving Noce a pat on the head, he said, "It means if we hold onto each other, we'll weather any storm."

Chapter Eighteen

DRIVING HOME FROM A PARTY IN THE SOLITUDE OF NIGHT, they spotted a frightened fawn standing in the center of the road. Steve slowed down and honked several times, but the fawn stood statue still. He pulled off to the side of the road and said, "Wait here, babe. If someone hits that animal out in the middle of nowhere, there'll be hell to pay."

"It's pitch black out there, Steve. Be careful."

Guided by the glow of the car's tail lights, he slowly walked back to the fawn and coaxed it to the edge of the road. When he reached out to touch the fawn's head, it leapt back and bounded into the thicket. Turning to jog back to the car, Steve caught his foot in a crevice, tripped, and landed on the jagged edge of the metal guardrail. Grabbing his side, he yelled out in agony and nearly passed out from the pain.

Dominic Rossi sat close to Jenna and urged her to drink some of his coffee while they waited in the emergency room for a doctor to update them on Steve's condition. Clare and Tony Gaone clung to each other to subdue their worry. After what seemed like hours of ex-rays and tests, the doctor pushed through the double doors and said, "He's a fortunate man. Besides some bruised muscles that should heal nicely, we want to keep an eye on the wound in his side. We'll hold him for another day to make sure an infection doesn't set in."

"Is he awake?" Jenna asked.

"The medication's making him groggy. We'll get him settled in a room, and you can stay with him as long as you want."

Jenna looked at Clare and said, "I should've never let him get out of the car."

Tony draped his arm on Jenna's shoulders and told her, "He was always bringing home strays and other critters. Rescuing that fawn doesn't surprise me." Drawing her closer, he said, "Stop blaming yourself. Accidents happen."

"I love him so much. I don't want to know what it's like to—"

Clare consoled, "Before you know it, he'll be home not following doctor's orders."

"Did anyone call Michael?" Jenna asked, her voice weak from fatigue.

Clare said, "Phil talked with him. He knows Steve's injuries aren't life-threatening, so he'll stay at school, and we'll keep him posted."

A nurse led them to Steve's room where Clare settled next to Tony on a small, gray couch. Turning to Dom and Rosie, Tony said, "No sense in all of us losing sleep. Go home and rest. We'll call if anything changes."

Jenna sat in a chair close to Steve's bed and kept watch over him.

Sharp sounds of hospital breakfast trays striking metal carts woke the Gaones from the soothing balm of sleep. The intermittent *bings*, paging doctors, and casual conversations between workers in the hallway reminded them that life goes on despite personal turmoil.

Jenna was sitting on the edge of Steve's bed massaging his hand when he opened his eyes, and asked, "How long have I been out?"

"Last night you saved the deer and tangled with a nasty guard rail."

He winced. "I remember." Holding his side, he winced again. "How long do I have to stay here?"

"If your temp is still normal through tomorrow, they'll release you."

He looked up at his mother first, then his father. "I'm sorry. I tried to do something good but . . ." He closed his eyes to block his emotions.

Tony patted his son's cheek and said, "Call Mike. Let him hear your voice, and tell him not to worry. Motioning with his head to the door, he told Clare, "I'm hungry. Let them talk while we get breakfast."

Clare palmed Steve's forehead to feel for a fever.

"Stop hovering, Mom. They have state of the art equipment to monitor temperatures."

Tony let out a laugh. "If your mother could lavish love on every kid like she does you and Phil, all those pharmaceutical companies that produce happy pills would go out of business."

"You love me enough to sneak me outta here, Mom?"

Planting a kiss on his forehead, Clare said, "Stay put. Infections can be nasty."

It was five in the morning, the day of Steve's discharge from the hospital, when an unlikely visitor stopped at the nurse's station. He requested special permission to visit Stephen Gaone before official visiting hours began. The day before, he had passed himself off as a business associate attempting to secure an appointment with Steve when Steve's secretary casually mentioned Steve's hospital stay.

Handsome and impeccably dressed, the visitor stood in the doorway of Steve's hospital room for several seconds before taking a seat in the corner of the still, dark room.

Steve woke to the shadowy figure struggling to subdue a hoarse cough. After a hard stare, Steve recognized the man.

"Must've been a helluva thunderstorm last night. I see the sewers overflowed into my room."

"I take it Jenna's told you about me?"

"With reluctance," Steve shot back.

Folding his handkerchief and tucking it in his blazer pocket, Ronan King said, "I apologize for waking you."

"Get out!"

Ronan crossed his legs and brushed his hand across his knee. "Not until I convince you to—"

"No! You don't have a stain's chance in a bleach factory of convincing me of anything."

Clearing his throat, Ronan said, "I'm dying, Mr. Gaone. I need Jenna to help me finalize my exit plan."

"You're delusional if you think Jenna will help you fictionalize a legacy." Through a fake yawn, he added, "Use some of mommy and daddy's money to hire a public relations firm to pretend people give a damn how you go out."

Business-like, he pressed Steve. "I know she doesn't need or want me in her life, but I need her. She's the only person I trust to execute my plan."

Steve let out an incredulous laugh. "The version I heard was she crowned you the *Ass-hole of New York*. And behold! Here you are dumping crap on me."

Ronan stood and stared at the flurry of activity outside the hospital window. He studied the pedestrians weaving in and out of traffic. After a screech or two from near misses, a glimmer of fight stirred in him. Turning to Steve, he asked, "Do your parents love you, Mr. Gaone?"

"Leave my parents out of this."

After a deliberate nod, Ronan continued saying, "My mother and father were swingers. It was a teenage guy's dream to have a steady supply of eager women inviting me to join the fun." Shrugging, he said, "The one drawback was the sound of my mother being handled by all those other men, knowing my father consented to it."

He turned to peer out the window and fixed his eyes on a woman holding a red umbrella standing beside a news stand. Swinging his eyes back to Steve who was staring at him with an aura of disbelief, Ronan said, "I knew the moment Jenna entered my bedroom, she was there because she loved me. What I didn't know . . . What I never learned was how to love her or any woman." His face expressed unmistakable amazement when he said, "I do know I cared more about Jenna than my dad cared about my mother. I made sure my frat brothers didn't take turns with her." Holding Steve's stare, he said, "That solitary act allows me to believe I'm not a complete monster." As if he still couldn't believe Carly's forgiveness, he added, "Then, I listened to a tape of a little girl full of love and forgiveness. She's waiting to love me in . . ." His voice cracked. "How does a man like me find a place in paradise?"

With a combination of curiosity and disgust, Steve asked, "Why are you dumping all this garbage on me? A priest wouldn't be able to stomach the sins you're spewing."

Without blinking, Ronan said, "Before this year's out, I'll be dead. There's a slim chance I can get my obituary to read more meaningfully than some kid's graffiti on a public bathroom stall." He let out a soft sigh. "No amount of money can erase the harm I've done over a lifetime of squalor." His face was drawn, his voice tired. "I'm not interested in recreating myself. I'd like to be a part of something real for once in my life, but I can't do it alone."

His eyes dropped when a nurse strolled in to check Steve's temperature and refresh his pitcher of water. When she exited, Ronan looked up, and said, "I don't have anywhere else to turn."

Steve pushed his hair back with his hand. "What the hell did you expect? How long did you think you could mess with people's lives before you ran up against someone or something that you couldn't buy?"

Heaping on more self-deprecation, Ronan told Steve, "If that was the worst of it, I'd be able to die in peace. When Jenna told me I had a daughter, my initial reaction was relief to hear she—"

Steve pointed at him and said, "I heard! You're the kind of person that makes me believe hell's not made of fire. It has to be a frigid place for one helluva cold, calculating, heart, don't you think?"

Ronan eyed Steve with a sinister grin and asked, "Did it ever occur to you that without cold-hearted bastards like me, judgmental knights in shining armor like you wouldn't get a chance to display your chivalry?" With a smirk, he added, "I've always been amused by holier than thou people who conveniently conceal their imperfections in and around other people's cesspools." He sat and crossed his leg over his knee. "As good as you are Gaone, Jenna's better." He pointed his finger at Steve and said, "I wish I had time to make lofty, sweeping reparation for my sins, but I don't. I need Jenna's forgiveness and—"

"Forgiveness? Why? Because you had to play a bad hand? The world abuses millions of people every day, and somehow they manage a level of decency." Punching an extra pillow before he stacked it behind his head, he said, "After mangling all sorts of lives, you slink in here and ask me to help you convince the most decent woman you ever screwed over to brush off how you broke her heart and came this close," he held his index finger and thumb close together, "to breaking her spirit. You want her to turn a blind eye to all the pain and suffering you caused her, so she can supply a positive spin on your hedonistic life?" His face red with anger, Steve hurled one last flogging. "There aren't words in any language that describe the brass balls you're carrying."

Ronan's adversarial stare pierced Steve for several moments. He coughed several times, wiped the beads of sweat from his forehead, and stuffed the white handkerchief into his coat pocket.

"I deserve your contempt, Gaone, but don't allow your ego to deny Jenna the satisfaction of hearing me apologize and acknowledge I hurt her."

Stunned by the prolific audacity of Ronan King's proposition, Steve wondered aloud, "I can't believe it took impending death to bring you to your knees."

Ronan turned his eyes to the busy street below. Horns honked as a child being dragged by his mother stumbled in traffic.

"There were always thick drapes and blinds on our windows throughout the house when I was growing up, but we made up for it in mirrors. There was never any meaningful interest or discussion about other people's lives." Sitting again, he brushed his knee several times, looked up, and said, "Jenna didn't mince words when she told me the only good I ever produced died the day our daughter died." He tugged at his cuff. "I shrugged it off until I heard Carly's voice on that tape several days after Jenna left New York."

Steve's voice carried admiration when he told Ronan, "Carly was a beautiful, valiant girl." Succumbing to sarcasm, he added, "The fact that she emerged from your gene pool remains a geneticist's riddle."

Disregarding Steve's flippant remark, Ronan stood and pleaded one last time. "Help me, Gaone. Help me reconcile to the only good thing in my life before I die. I feel the frigid force of hell from where I stand." Clearing his throat, he said, "Where else in God's universe does He assign a man who's responsible for two abortions and the callous indifference of his daughter's death?"

A wave of remorse washed over Steve. Posturing with slight consideration, he asked, "So, what's your grand plan?"

Business-like, Ronan explained, "I pooled my estate under one umbrella. I'd like to name it *The Carly McCoy Foundation.* The facility and funds will serve as a resource to help abused children overcome some of the obstacles they face." Jutting his chin as if ready to take a hit, he said, "I wish I could've managed my life with as much heart as some people who've experienced emotional and spiritual deficits. Maybe Jenna and I would've . . ." Gently shrugging, he said, "I know she loves and respects you. You're all I have to sway her."

Piercing him with a cold stare, Steve said, "The Great Wall of China would've been easier to dismantle than the barrier she built around herself because of you."

"The wall would've been impenetrable had I not removed her from my frat house that night."

Steve laid his head back on the pillows and stared at the antagonist before him. Running his hand through his hair, he asked, "What's Plan B if I refuse to cooperate?"

Subduing a short coughing spell and inconspicuously depositing phlegm in a hanky, he said, "There is no Plan B. My estate is in place to form a foundation to aid abused children. I need you to convince Jenna that my intention is legitimate so the McCoys will allow the foundation to bear Carly's name."

"What makes you believe Jen and I give a damn about how you spend eternity?"

Before Ronan turned to walk away, he handed Steve his card, and said, "If you didn't have a heart underneath all that warranted hostility, Jenna wouldn't be yours."

Chapter Nineteen

"SUPPER'S WARM ON THE STOVE," CLARE TOLD JENNA AND STEVE as she grabbed her coat and stood at the door. "I hope I beat the traffic. Dad and I are meeting friends for dinner."

"Scram, old lady," Steve teased, jumping up faster than he should have to hug his mother goodbye. Wincing at the pain in his side, he nearly toppled onto the coffee table.

Shooting him a stern stare, Clare warned, "Stay put, Stephen. What's it going to take to keep you from landing in the hospital with a broken neck?"

Steve grabbed his mother and said, "I owe you, *Mommy Dearest*."

Gently guiding him back to the couch, she said, "Maybe you would've been less oppositional had I used that psycho Joan Crawford's parenting techniques. Show more gratitude and buy me tickets to see *Cirque du Soleil*."

"My parents plan to see the show in Vegas next month," Jenna told her. "I'll get you tickets."

Clare pointed at Steve. "I'm calling Rosie as soon as I get home. In the meantime, try to stay in one piece."

The dishwasher loaded with after supper dishes whirred as Jenna plopped ice cubes in her ginger ale. Steve shuffled alongside her to the den where he eased himself beside her on the couch. She took a sip of her drink then gently snuggled close to him. Massaging her hand, he vacillated before broaching the topic of Ronan's proposition.

"I had an unlikely visitor in the hospital this morning."

Puzzled, she asked, "Who'd bother you that early? I was there by eight."

Without mincing words, he said, "Ronan King."

Jenna's jaw dropped. She snapped her eyes shut for several seconds, then jumped up. "Tell me this is your worst joke ever, Stephen."

Holding both hands up, palms facing her, he said, "You might find his request commendable, even for him."

Covering her mouth with her hands, she talked through her fingers. "That man's incapable of being decent." Pointing at Steve, she said, "I want him to stay out of my life."

"Soon enough," Steve told her with a deadly stare.

Absorbed by her anger, the full weight of his comment escaped her. She shot back, "A few months back, the sound of his name nauseated you. Now, you're his patron saint interceding on his behalf?" Shaking her head, she said, "No! He walked away. Now I want him to stay away."

He patted the couch and said, "It won't hurt to hear the whole story before you decide not to help him."

Flipping her hair back hard, she blurted out another emphatic, "No!" She turned to walk away, but he yanked her arm with more force than he intended causing her to tumble close to him onto the couch.

Holding his side to subdue a sharp pain, he clenched his teeth, and said, "Right now my body aches, but that guy's been racked with some pretty heavy stressors all his life."

Wide-eyed, she asked, "So, after one conversation with him, he's convinced you to dismiss the pain he heaped on others?" Shaking her head, she told him, "Don't ask me to give anything Ronan has to say my attention."

A crooked smile played on his lips. "How about giving what I have to say some attention?"

Gently nudging him with her elbow, she burrowed deeper into the couch, and said, "What Ronan deserves is one of the hottest places in hell. He's enough to make Lucifer sick of sin."

Pulling back, Steve sang, "Round and round the cauldron go; from Jenna's cold heart let mercy flow."

Defending herself, she countered, "Don't try to make me feel guilty for withholding sympathy for him, Steve. He made me lose my baby."

More seriously, Steve said, "He may have found a way for both of you to hold onto Carly, even share her with thousands of deserving people. He wants to keep Carly's memory alive with a facility, a foundation and scholarships for abused kids." His voice carried sympathy when he added, "He'll be dead in six months, Jen. My guess is he's trying to stave off that horrible date with the devil you hyperbolized a moment ago."

Her mouth gaped. "He's really dying?"

Steve nodded.

A smirk crossed her lips. "God really does mete out even handed justice."

Surprised by her uncharacteristic mean spirit, he furrowed his brow, and asked, "How's your reaction to his impending death any different than his reaction to Carly's death?"

"Carly was his innocent child."

"If childhood innocence is mitigating, maybe you owe it to him to hear the rest of his story." Sitting sideways, he looked straight at her, and said, "Unlike Carly, Ronan never had a chance to be innocent."

Mired in her obstinacy, she pointed at Steve, and said, "I owe Ronan nothing." Piercing him with adamant eyes, she said, "The only reason why I'm still listening to you guilt me into believing I have to be the one who intercedes on Ronan's behalf is because I love you."

Playing with her fingers, he said, "Fair enough. Love for me keeps you listening, but don't let hate for him blind you to the truth." Pulling her close, he told her, "He understands that you bore the only good part of him. He wants to keep that good alive. He's not seeking any publicity, no fanfare."

She pulled away, covered her mouth with her hands, and said, "My God! He plans to use his dead child as a get out of hell card." Dumbfounded, she asked, "Don't you see? It's always about him."

"I don't know, Jen. He accepted responsibility for two abortions." Judging that she didn't believe him, he pulled himself up off the couch, looked down at her, and said, "As if that confession wasn't humbling enough, he explained from where his hatred of women stemmed."

"That's no surprise," Jenna said. "He hates himself."

Steve's brow rose. "Ever since grade school, he had a front row seat to his prim and proper parents by day swinging with other couples by night. Sometimes the parties got out of hand. He was a confused kid who found it difficult to understand why his father let other guys play with his mother."

Narrowing her eyes, she asked, "Ronan told you that?"

"They even dragged him into the fun a few times. Welcome to the world of misogyny makers."

She shook her head and said, "What happened between us in college was consensual, not brutal in the least."

He took a drink from his water bottle and said, "What his frat brothers planned to do with you wouldn't have been as wholesome." His eyes searched her face. "The love you expressed moved him to love you the only way he knew how. Ronan got you out of that house before those guys could hurt you."

Stunned by the revelation, she sat speechless.

"I worked through every scenario, Jenna. I don't see what he'd gain by exposing his depravity. His foundation will forward goodness all the way around. How is it wrong for people to remember him in a positive way if he's responsible for achieving something necessary and good?"

Gaining composure, she asked, "How do you know he's really dying?"

"Was he coughing when you met him in New York?"

"He hacked away several times."

"He has lung cancer that's spread throughout his body. Doctors give him six months at most."

Sinking deeper into the couch, she said, "After everything I've gone through, you want me to help save this jackass's soul?" She closed her eyes and wondered aloud, "Will God ever stop punishing me for my one night of indiscretion?"

"Maybe God's giving you an opportunity to transform chaos into order."

"What kind of god orchestrates misery and disorder in the first place?" she asked.

"We're the ones who wander off in wrong directions." He let out a laugh. "Think of God as a universal GPS, always recalculating when we lose direction. Sooner or later, He gets us to where He wants us to be."

"And where are we supposed to be, Steve? Frankly, I can use a few roadside rests along the way of watching everyone I know suffering because of my directionally challenged life."

Eyeing her, he said, "Ronan suffered, too."

She jumped up. "I won't let you equate Ronan's suffering with my parents' and the McCoys' suffering. If he would've possessed a thread of decency, we wouldn't be having this conversation."

Disappointed in her reaction, he grabbed her hand and ordered, "Sit down and stop being obtuse. We've all suffered, and we've all caused our share of suffering."

Resigning herself, she sat back down.

Softening, he said, "I'm not denying the chaos in our lives, but don't turn your back on opportunities to redirect the chaos into something good."

Palming her chest, she asked, "Why me?"

"All I know is Ronan King seemed destined for damnation until your love stirred some level of goodness in him, and from that goodness came an even greater good called Carly McCoy."

With hope in her voice, Jenna asked, "Are you saying Carly was conceived in love, at least as close to love as Ronan could manage?"

"He protected you then, and he trusts you now."

The idea that she conceived her baby in love softened her. With less hostility, but still confused, she asked, "What now?"

Steve held up Ronan's business card and said, "Find out what his next move is before he meets his maker."

"I can't believe I have to help Ronan King get good with God."

"Maybe it's time we all get good with God." Through a wide yawn, he added, "Since you're contemplating helping wounded men in your life, help me up the stairs."

Lying in his bed, Stephen rested his head on two fluffed up pillows as music from the CD player downstairs filtered to the bedroom. Grappling with his covers, he stared at her, his eyes growing large and bright.

"Now what?" she asked with mock irritation.

"It just occurred to me that if you help your ex, guess who'll be the happiest of all?"

"Straightening his sheet twisted up in the blanket, she told him, "All I know is every cab driver in New York will have a fatwa on me by dusk once they find out I helped that disgusting creature."

"They won't know you helped him, but Carly will." He massaged her shoulders and said, "Remember how she described everyone being together again in heaven? That girl's jumping up and down squealing, 'Oh my gosh!' because her dad loves both of you."

Jenna's eyes rolled over him in wonderment. "There's not a man alive who has better ability to focus on the good in every fragmented situation that people face." Reminding hm, she said, "There was a time when Ronan King threatened you. Now, you're encouraging me to see the good in him, even save him." She kissed his cheek. "You must feel confident in my love."

"That's more credit than I deserve, Jen. I struggled with this one. The temptation to disregard a dying man's plea gnawed at me."

"You weren't going to tell me?"

Quiet at first, he folded his arms across his chest, and said, "He was your first love. Someone beautiful came out of . . ." Unable to verbalize the fear of losing her, his boyish eyes begged her to love him back.

She gently picked at the blanket and admitted, "I was crazy about Ronan once." Studying Steve's face, she said, "I was full of immature emotions." Pressing her forehead onto his, she whispered, "Lying in your arms is more sacramental; I belong here." She let out a laugh saying, "The GPS God guided me here. Besides," she said nonchalantly, "the only other man who hasn't dismissed me from his heart after I displayed mounds of imperfections and ingratitude is my father." Caressing his cheek, she told him, "A first love is like a footnote in a long document of life. You're my last love, the thesis, the theme, the reason for every other word, sentence, paragraph, and page in my document of life."

An easy sigh escaped him. Tapping her chest with his index finger, he said, "You owned me the moment you sashayed into that conference room and whipped that Banshee head of hair all over your sexy, bare shoulders."

"I never sashay," she countered, feigning insult. "One look at you and I praised God for parent/teacher conferences."

Clasping his hands behind his head, he said, "I thought you didn't like God."

"What gave you that absurd idea?"

"Your bi-polar reaction every time we discuss a deity."

Philosophizing, she said, "I've been fighting with God ever since first grade when Sister Mary Theresa warned us to stop asking questions because the universe holds all kinds of mysteries that will never be ours to know." With a shrug, she said, "I hate not knowing."

"Sister Mary Theresa was right."

"I know," she told him as she tucked him in, "but I always find myself pushing the boundaries."

Playing with his hair, she told him, "I'll talk to Ronan, but if he provokes me . . ."

"Think positive thoughts."

"Admit it, Stephen. Ronan would make Jesus, Gandhi, and Martin Luther King want to rough him up in a back alley."

Pressing his hand over her mouth, he asked, "How can you tolerate Sam's incessant nagging, yet cast an avalanche of insults on a dying man asking for a favor?"

"Ronan hurt me; Sam didn't." Narrowing her eyes, she said, "Time to get some rest, cowboy, before I ask you to explain why you're so understanding of Ronan's loss of innocence, yet Samantha Kind's damaged existence repels you."

Blinking his tired eyes, he said, "It's one of those mysteries beyond our understanding that Sister Mary Theresa was talking about."

Snuggling close to him, she said, "I wonder what Sam and Ronan would've been like if their parents would've sacrificed for them."

Resting her head on his chest, they lay together soothed by the sound of soft music and the synchronized beating of their hearts. Dozing off, he mumbled, "They would've kept the water outta the ship."

Chapter Twenty

HER WEDDING ONLY A MONTH AWAY, JENNA WORE AN AIR of confidence as she followed the hostess to where Ronan stood to greet her in an upscale, New York restaurant.

He said softly, "I wasn't sure you'd come."

"Steve convinced me," she said, eyeing him with guarded curiosity.

Playing with the edge of his napkin, he said, "I envy him."

Her genuine smile calmed him. She sipped some water and said directly, "I'm sorry for what happened to you; I would've treated—"

Holding up his hand, he said, "Please don't. You, of all people, owe me no apologies. I nearly ruined your life." After a quick scan of the dining area, he came back to her and said, "I ruined a lot of lives, and for that, I have hell to pay." He picked up his glass and took a small gulp of water. "I'm sorry is woefully inadequate, but necessary." He looked away for a moment and stared at the waitress clearing off the table several feet from them. Turning back to Jenna, he cleared his throat and said, "Tell me about Carly."

Jenna grew misty. "I only knew her briefly before she died." Her eyes fell to the table. Using a napkin to catch the tears before they ran to her cheeks, she looked up and forced a smile. "She had your dimpled chin and your charisma. Only she was more optimistic."

Satisfaction crossed his face. He sat back and said, "I don't blame you for distrusting my motives. I've always pretended not to be a scared bastard. Dying's forcing me to admit the only person I fooled was myself."

"We all find ways to convince ourselves that we're better than we really are," she consoled. "Regardless, the foundation's a wonderful way to remember Carly and help so many emotionally wounded children. The McCoys are good people. I'll talk to them." She swirled her drink and teased, "The first thing Carly wanted to know was if you were a jerk."

He pulled back and coughed several times. "Spare my shattered ego the details of that conversation."

Searching his face, she said, "I owed her the truth. I told her you were the handsomest guy on campus, but you weren't ready to get serious about life." Her eyes dropped when she said apologetically, "I told her I never gave you a chance to know about her."

When Ronan whispered Jenna's name, she looked up. He said, "Thank you. You spared your child . . . our child needless pain." With a hint of bitterness, he added, "That's more than my mother did for me."

She nodded.

Letting out a sarcastic laugh, he said, "I dreamed that my last conversation with my mother would offer some closure. I fantasized her saying something like, 'I never meant to screw up your life,' and then she'd die in my forgiving arms." With a bitter edge to his voice, he said, "Even on her deathbed, she couldn't muster any kindness. When I asked her why they partied, she told me, 'It was the only way I could keep your father interested.'" Clearing his throat, he apologized and sipped some wine.

For several quiet moments, he eyed a couple who sat across the aisle from them. Turning back to Jenna, he said, "Meeting with you after all these years and listening to Carly's voice on that tape made me realize the price I paid for wrapping myself up in hate."

As Ronan coughed hard for several seconds, Jenna stared at the bottle of wine to give him a moment to catch his breath. Raising her eyes, she said, "Carly was the best of us." Smiling, she assured him, "That girl was convinced that you couldn't be that bad if I loved you. I guess neither of us is that bad, because she loved both of us."

His eyes glistened. "I'm thankful you were wise enough and strong enough never to give a frightened, angry," he fought for the right words, "emotionally challenged man-child like me the power to cause her misery."

Searching his tired face, she said, "One reason I love Stephen Gaone is he teaches me to grab hold of whatever shred of good there is in every horrible scenario life throws in our path." With an air of whimsy, she added, "Steve's always creating life-saving devices out of debris that floats his way." Several seconds of silence passed between them before she said, "In all the wreckage we've been wading through, we're fortunate that we can latch onto the memory of a little girl that promises to bring us to a place of peace."

Caught off guard by her sincere determination to save him, he lowered his eyes and sat in awkward silence. Jenna's willingness to forgive him gently washed over his grimy soul when she said, "We all suffered, Ronan, partly because others mistreated us, partly because we made bad decisions." He looked up with pleading eyes. Holding his gaze, she said, "We may not be where we need to be, but at least we're not where we used to be, stuck in our fear and hardened hearts." Digging into her purse, she pulled out one of Carly's heart-shaped stones. Gently running her fingers over the treasured rock, she asked him, "Will you do me a favor?"

He brightened. "I owe you that much."

"The only way I can finally let Carly go is to know you'll be with her." Dabbing her eyes with a napkin, she said, "She already loves you. Her eyes won't lie." She slid the stone across the marble table. "This was from her *heart* collection. Carry it with you. Tell her she'll be in my heart forever."

He closed his hand around the heart formation and raised it to his lips. Studying her face, he said, "I wish I could've believed someone as wonderful as you loved me. Maybe . . ." He turned his head, coughed, and motioned for the waitress to fill their water glasses. The music played louder as the restaurant emptied after the noon rush.

Jenna studied his face before she reached over and tapped the back of his hand. "No more pedaling backwards. Let's step away from the sadness right here, right now."

"How does a person walk away from a lifetime of emptiness and pain?"

"It's not easy, but if we can find one person who promises to wait for us and renew our lives with love, it's worth trading the pain for the promise."

Jenna and Ronan lingered outside the restaurant. People rushing back to work inadvertently bumped into them as they managed a long good-bye. Ronan leaned close and whispered, "Others were opiates, dulling my senses, my sense. You've given me a reason to live the rest of my life clear-headed with anticipation."

A second before he slipped into his cab, she called his name.

He turned to her.

Blowing him a kiss, she called out, "For Carly."

Ronan snatched the kiss from mid-air and palmed his chest. As Jenna watched his cab wind its way through a colorful sea of moving metal, she envisioned a flickering lamp undulating on gentle waves carrying his soul to a place of peace. The sorrow she bore for much of her life slipped away with him. She raised her eyes to heaven, but her phone pre-empted her prayer.

"I wish I was dead," Sam blurted out. Bloated on bourbon, she asked, "How come men have ta be scum?" Whispering, she told Jenna, "I invited one over last night." Growing shrill, she cried, "And he hurt me."

Rolling her eyes, Jenna asked, "Where'd you meet this guy?"

Jenna held the phone away from her ear as Sam yelled, "Why's that matter? I thought he was gonna be nice, but he's like . . ." She garbled her words, "He'slike alltherest."

"What'd he do?"

Following a long, guttural groan, Sam whimpered, "I really tried. I tried to be a good girl and . . . and to make him . . . to make him happy, butI . . . butI . . . butI . . . I vomited. Oh God, Jen. I threw up all over him." Her sobs grew louder. "He shoved me." More lucid, she said, "He shoved me, and he called me ugly names." After another crying spell, she said, "I just want someone to hold me. All they ever want . . . You know what they always want." Sounding like a muffled fog horn, she blew her nose and settled into child-like whimpers. "He was touching me all over. Touched me like my daddy used to." After a short pause, her cold detached voice said, "I wanna kill them over and over and over again."

"You're not a killer, Sam. Besides, you can't pick some drunk up in a bar and expect—"

"Here we go again. Blame me, go ahead and blame me!" she yelled. "Is it a crime . . . to want . . . to want someone to be nice to me? If I don't invite people over, I don't talk to anyone or see anyone except store clerks for weeks at a time. I'm notta bad person; I'm a good girl." Her voice turned sinister saying, "But sometimes . . . Sometimes I don't wannabe good. Sometimes . . ." She paused to blow her nose. "Sometimes I wanna kill every single man I—"

Listening to Sam's incessant complaints forced Jenna's head into a tailspin. She watched passers-by dodge cars forcing them to a screeching stand-still. Horns blared at careless pedestrians who yelled back with indignation.

More irritated than usual, Jenna said, "Slow down, Sam. We talked for over an hour day before yesterday."

"Oh, and that's supposed to make up for all the other lonely days in my life? How many people hugged you in the last day and a half?"

Pacifying her conscience, Jenna fidgeted in guilt for several moments before she diverted the conversation saying, "Guess what? I met someone in New York who understands what you experienced. Do you remember me back in college talking about Ronan King?"

Sam paused and recalled Ronan's name more quickly than Jenna thought possible.

Put off by Jenna's choice to visit New York instead of paying her a visit, Sam said with exaggeration, "I can't *beeelieeeve* you made time for that pig. Heee screeewed you. Heee walked out on you, but you chose to visit *him*, not me!"

"He's dying, Sam."

"So what!" she yelled, her voice oozing venom. "People've been tryin' to kill me since the day I was born. Don't see any first responders knocking down my door. He's a brich . . . a rich bastard. Tell'im to hire servants to help his sorry ass. I can't believe you chose him over me. That's a lap . . . a real slap in the face. You really hurt me, Jenna."

Ignoring Sam's accusatory tirade, Jenna said, "His mother abused him when he was a kid. You distrust men; he doesn't trust women."

A dramatic gasp escaped Sam. "His mother hurt him?" Whispering like a child petrified to get caught divulging a family secret, she said, "He should've killed her. When they hurt you like that . . . you're allowed . . . You should be allowed ta kill them."

"That's silly talk, Sam. Besides, the people who hurt you and Ronan are dead. Stop giving them power to hold you from a brighter future."

Sam screamed, "They're not just any people; they were my mother and father! They were monsters. They didn't love . . . They hurt me so much." She let loose a torrent of tears. After the cathartic release, she said between sniffles, "I wanna hold him, tell him . . . Tell him it'sgonna be okay. It's gonna be okay, isn't it, Jen?"

"You'll both be okay. He knows his time is short; he's setting his affairs in order. I forgave him because I understand—"

"You forgave him? It wasn't his fault! Our mothers treated us like white ravens. They pecked and pecked and pecked at us. They refused to love us; they killed the good in us. He should've stabbed . . ." Her voice lowered to a whisper. "He should've killed her like I . . ." Raising her voice again to a screaming crescendo, she said, "People should be begging him . . . on their knees begging him for forgiveness!"

Sam's screech forced Jenna to hold the phone away from her ear. With a calm but firm voice, Jenna told Sam, "I can't bear another moment of your tirade. Calm down or I'm ending this discussion."

After several moments of silence, Sam asked with a pout, "Who cares anyway?"

Jenna's voice softened. "They hurt you, but they didn't kill the good in you. You're a wonderful person. Besides, Ronan admits he hurt me. I forgave him. We're okay."

With anger induced sobriety, her voice was deliberate and clear. "Oooh, there's Miss Priss, passing out forgiveness again like Christ Almighty. Get it through your thick skull that *he* doesn't need your forgiveness. He didn't do anything wrong! People should apologize to him! He's the victim! We're the victims!" she screeched. Lowering her voice one decibel, she screamed, "They screwed us! They put us in roasting pans and turned the oven on to five hundred goddamn degrees and placed bets to see what temperature I'd start screaming to high heaven! When my mother found out, you think she got me the hell away from that psychotic bastard? Oooh nooo! Instead, one day when we were fighting, she told me to shut my mouth about what he did to me because he could go to jail and how would we get money to live, and you wonder why I can't trust people? Why I hate hate hate men? He should've never ever apologized to you. I hate him for apologizing to you!" Her heaving sobs unleashed servile misery.

Unable to curb her frustration, Jenna said, "Look Sam, I had a rough day, so—"

Sam's voice turned cold and cutting. "Poor baby. Stop the world and let Jenna Rossi jump off. She had a damn rough day!" As bourbon filled her glass, she said, "You jet-set to New York to have a fling with an old boyfriend while your new boyfriend sits home twiddling his thumbs waiting for you to come home and marry him, and you're whining about a rough day? Let me describe what a rough day really is, Miss Priss. Live with a mother who grabs . . . She grabbed me by my hair and dragged me kicking and screaming to my stinkin', drunken father because she was too tired to service him. Watch your father come at you with a gun to blow a hole through your chest and have his blood splatter in your face when you shoot him because it's the only way to save your miserable, stinkin' life. Try spendin' most of your day every single day wishing you could kill him over and over again cuz . . . cuz . . . it felt so . . ." she stopped short and asked, "Who cares anyway?"

Still sitting on a bench outside the restaurant, some passers-by stared at Jenna as she palmed her face. Interrupting Sam's sobs, she said, "I can't believe you whipped yourself into frenzy. No one blames you or Ronan for what happened to you as children."

Tiring herself out, Sam's voice slurred saying, "Then why'd that one dumbcop seep sayin' . . . I mean keep sayin' 'somethin's not right'? Everyone else believes me."

"Cops are suspicious by nature. If they thought you murdered your father, you'd be in jail."

"Right," Sam said with new-found confidence. "But there's no statute of limitation on murder, so I always . . . I always have ta worry 'bout that one dumb cop." As an afterthought, she said, "Maybe someday his car'll explode."

"Geez, Sam. Death isn't the answer to every problem."

"So, now yer defendin' the cop? My psychiatrist warned me about you. She told me to hang up on you when you refuse to support me."

Building a strong dislike for Sam's analyst from the moment Sam revealed some of the disturbing, unconventional methods the doctor practiced, Jenna shot back, "I've been your friend ever since kindergarten. You've only known that quack for several months. Every time I answer my phone and subject myself to your manipulative abuse, I'm supporting you. I love you, Sam, but frankly, I'm tired of hearing about what your second-rate psychiatrist thinks I should be doing for you when you're paying big bucks for her advice twice a week, and I . . ." She stopped short. Ice clinked in a glass, followed by the muffled sound of the receiver being fumbled in Sam's drunken hands. Then dead silence.

Jenna shoved her phone into her purse, looked up to heaven with defiance, and threatened, "One of these days I'll just let it keep ringing."

Chapter Twenty-One

"WE NEED TO GET GOING. THEY WANT US FOR PICTURES before the ceremony." Staring at his father who was in front of a mirror straightening his tie, Mike added, "Uncle Phil called. They're on their way with the limo. Jenna's gonna think you jilted her."

He turned to his son and said, "Isn't the groom the one who's supposed to be nervous?" Motioning for Mike to sit, he said, "Let's talk before we get lost in the crowd."

Mike sat on the edge of the bed. "Something wrong?"

"No. This time, it's all right." He stared at his son for several seconds before saying, "I want you to know how meaningful you've made my life."

Mike began to fidget. "Dad, you don't have to—"

"Yes, I do." He pulled up a chair and straddled it backwards. "Remember when I was getting close to Karen?"

Mike nodded. "Nonna told me why you broke it off."

Comically pulling away, Steve asked, "How'd she know?"

"She spotted some ripped up boarding school pamphlets in the garbage. She told me it was a sure sign that you loved me more than you loved any woman."

"I can't believe Nonna knew Karen planned to send you away, and she still let her live." Rolling his eyes, he said, "That lady dodged a bullet."

Mike laughed.

Steve stood, looked down at his son, and said, "One reason why I love Jenna is she never tried to usurp your place in my heart." Palming his chest, he said, "You will forever be right here, and I will forever be grateful to your mother for sharing you with me."

Mike stood, embraced his father, and said, "On some of Mom's good days, she'd tell me that someday you were going to be my best friend."

Steve's eyes blurred.

Mike extended a hanky and teased, "I was saving this for Jenna."

Steve grabbed the handkerchief, brushed his cheek, and said, "Men cry, too, Michael."

Mike admitted, "I've done my share. But I hooked you up with the hottest lady in town, so dry your eyes and go get married before she marries someone else and gives you something really to cry about."

Steve flashed a bright smile. "I owe you big time."

After a quick fist bump, Mike said, "Call it even."

The wedding festivities waned around midnight. Steve swept Jenna up in his arms and carried her over the threshold of their quiet home. He playfully pushed her up against the bedroom wall, fumbled the zipper to her gown, and said, "Hallelujah! We've made it to the procreation free zone. Let the fireworks be—"

She planted a long, lingering kiss on his lips, and said, "Don't light that Roman candle just yet, cowboy. Our flight leaves in an hour and a half. We'll have to delay the pyrotechnics for several hours."

"Change the flight," he said, gently tugging her toward the bed.

Wiggling from his grip, she slipped out of her gown, grabbed her jeans, and said, "We'd have to change all the hotel and entertainment arrangements. Let's avoid the hassle and just make the flight. She tossed his jeans to him, and said, "I promise to make it up to you."

He dropped on the bed and stared at the ceiling. Covering his face with his hands, he pleaded, "Tell me you're jesting, Mrs. Gaone."

Zipping up her pants with one hand, she gently swatted his leg with the other, and said, "Let's go." With an infectious smile, she coaxed, "You'll look better wearing those jeans instead of that frown. I'll drive."

After loading their luggage in the car, he said, "Toss me the keys."

She dangled them in front of him and said, "I know a shortcut."

"There's no shortcut to the airport, Jen."

"Hop in and learn, cowboy."

She drove the speed limit on the freeway until she sped past the exit that clearly designated the route to the airport.

"Slow down, Lady Leadfoot. That was our exit you covered in dust."

"I'm taking a different route."

With a hint of exasperation in his voice, he said, "I told you, there's no other way. Pull over and give me the keys."

Focusing on the road ahead, she told him, "Trust me, Stephen, my detour's better."

Shooting her a sideways glance, he asked, "When did it become a detour?"

Before she could answer, the car gently began to rock on rough terrain familiar to him. "Why in the names of Buddha, Mohammad, and Jesus Christ are we headed toward my cabin?"

"Our cabin," she corrected him. "I didn't want to upset you, so—"

"Too late," he said, his voice loaded with sarcasm. "Won't this shortcut, detour, or whatever you're calling it, make us miss our flight?"

"Don't be mad," she said screwing up her face, bracing for his protest, "but I already moved our flight to tomorrow afternoon."

"Then why couldn't we . . . Never mind," he snapped.

Feeling his muscles tighten, he averted a fight by laying his head back, closing his eyes, and seething in silence.

Fifteen minutes later, Jenna pulled up to the cabin porch. She jumped out of the car, raised her hands high over her head, and proclaimed, "Our life begins here!"

A swell of excitement returned as Steve unloaded the luggage they needed, He told her, "Let's pass on a fire; the night's sultry."

He eagerly followed her toward the bedroom when she stopped, turned, and placed her hand on his chest. "You stay here."

He raised his hands high over his head and said, "As you wish."

When she disappeared into the bedroom, he sprawled on the carpet in front of the fireplace and rested his eyes. Creaking floor boards alerted him to the presence of his bride wearing a canary yellow net top, the kind that covers a bathing suit. One hard blink confirmed the bathing suit was missing. His eyes followed her as she glided across the room. She caught the doorknob, hesitated, and asked seductively, "Do you want to come with me?"

His heart raced as he sprang to his feet. "Out there? In the dark?"

"There's a full moon, and we have this," she said, raising the lantern to her chest. She opened the door and gave a slight motion with her head.

The moonlight surfed the contours of her body as she gingerly situated the lantern at the edge of the dock. Silver-crested ripples gently lapped at the shoreline. Every movement she made, every look she threw his way heightened passion in him. Before he could reach her, she lifted her arms, slipped off her top, and playfully flung it in his face. The intoxicating scent of her lingered in the air as he watched in mild shock how she called out, "Jenna Rossi's jumping in!" She leaped high into the air and plunged into the water with a splash, jetting deep into blackness. Seconds later, her head broke through the surface with a softer splash. She quickly wiped her face with her hands and yelled, "Mrs. Stephen Gaone is coming out!" Her glistening face coupled with her playful laughter filled the quiet night and beckoned him. Stripping with lightning speed, he dove in.

From toe to lips, his body glided upward alongside hers, breaking the surface with wild desire. Treading water in time with her, he wrapped one arm around her waist and pulled her close saying, "In my wildest dreams, I never would've guessed you'd make this scene a reality."

She began to explain, "I want to be Mrs. Stephen Gaone body and soul," when a slithering sensation along the inside of her leg seized her with panic. She let loose a blood curdling scream and flailed her arms in a desperate attempt to reach the dock. "Something's crawling on me!" she yelled. Thrashing uncontrollably, she screamed, "Get it off me!" With one heave, she was out of the water. She crossed her arms over her chest and flew up the path to the cabin, yelling, "Kill it, Steve! Kill it!"

Panting like a lion in pursuit of his prey, he caught up to her and said, "Calm down, Jenna. I'm the only animal chasing you." He wiggled his fingers in front of her face then slid his hand up the inside of her leg.

Sucking in a breath of surprise, she covered her mouth with her hands. "You pawed me on purpose?"

"Some people call it foreplay," he said, planting a kiss on her neck.

Giddy with excitement, she gently shoved his shoulder, and said, "I could've died of shock in that lake."

"I could've died as monster bait while you escaped."

"Oh my gosh! I left you there to die!" Playing with the hairs on his chest, she asked, "How can I make it up to you?"

Her pseudo-dramatic apology heightened excitement in him. Swooping her up, he carried her into the bedroom. "No more detours, Mrs. Gaone. We've arrived."

Isolated from the concerns of society, they played together. She arched her frame as his hands and lips canvassed the more mysterious, sensitive terrain of her body.

"The wait to love you without barriers was worth it," he whispered in a breathy voice.

She folded her hands behind her head, seductively crossed one leg over her knee, and asked, "Now that the siege has ended, what does my handsome liege plan to do with me?"

Her suggestive pose heated up the blood coursing through his veins. "I plan to give you everything in life you've ever wanted."

"All I ever wanted was to fall in love with a man whose heart would love me at my worst." Rolling off the bed, she said, "I guess we're done here."

Adrenaline surged through his body as he pulled her back. "Not so fast, Rossi."

"Gaone," she corrected him.

She laid her head back on the pillow, gave him an innocent wide-eyed stare, and asked, "You have something more?"

The lantern cast long shadows over the room as he bridged her body with his arms. He let out a low, lusty laugh and said, "I thought when this moment came, I'd pounce on you, drive myself to wild ecstasy, and ravish you beyond—"

Narrowing her eyes, she gently shoved his chest with her knee. "I thought Gaone men don't lie."

His eyes widened. "I'm trying to be romantic, here." Grabbing her leg, he caressed it up to her inner thigh and said, "Forgive me for being shocked that you passed up Hawaii to skinny dip with me in the lake at midnight."

Running her knee back and forth across his chest, her voice sensuously sang, "Sounds like a delay tactic. All that brawny bragging you did since the day I met you was bound to catch up with you sooner or later."

Her playful taunt incited his pounding heart. Unable to contain his passion, he tilted his head, grinned, and with one stroke of his hand, he brushed her leg aside and swept her up in his arms. Just as quickly, he leaned forward and pressed his body hard onto hers. She happily surrendered as he rocked in rhythmic motion coaxing soft groans from her. Pushing her over the brink to ecstasy, she radiated a peace about her when she whispered breathlessly, "I stand corrected."

Nibbling her earlobe, he whispered, "My lady's lying."

She let out a soft laugh and played with his pun. "I never knew lying could make a person feel so alive."

His warm breath on her neck excited her as he planted tender kisses down to her chest and back up to her ear. He whispered, "I never wanted to live a lie, but lying here with you makes life worth living."

Chapter Twenty-Two

"BELIEVE IN GOD?" THE CHURCH MARQUEE ASKED. "SAY *AMEN* and claim a miracle!"

Samantha barreled down the main street in town, weaving back and forth across the road. Ignoring the stop sign at the intersection, she zigzagged to miss a semi rumbling by, jumped the curb, and landed on the front lawn of the church. She pushed the car door open and tumbled onto the grass. She stood and staggered toward the marquee. Clasping her hands, she prayed, "IbelieveinGod! IbelieveinGod! IbelieveinGod!"

She waited several seconds, anticipating the transformational force of the miracle the marquee promised. God's angels remained silent. Her agitated eyes scanned the yard and moved outward to the street, but the world lying before her was devoid of comfort. She turned to the marquee. This time she repeated her words louder and more distinctly, tracing the letters behind the glass with her fingertip.

"I . . . be . . . lieve . . . in . . . God! I . . . be . . . lieve . . . in . . . God! I . . . be . . . lieve . . . in . . . God!"

She stood at attention, barely breathing, piercing the marquee with a cold stone stare. She gave God ample time to perform the miracle He promised.

"I believe in God. I *really* believe in you, God," she whispered in her most fervent voice.

Her eyes focused like lasers on the marquee as anger swelled in her like boiling milk rising in a pot over high heat. She pulled at her hair and screamed, "I did what you told me to do! I always did what they told me to do!" She kicked some stones into the air and demanded, "Where's my miracle?" Escalating to frenzy, she whirled around, picked up a large rock, and flung it into the marquee. She slammed the broken glass several times with her bare fist and cried, "Die, you liar! Die! Die! Die!"

An alarmed motorist called 911.

When paramedics arrived, they found Samantha groveling on the church lawn licking the blood dripping from her shredded hand. She lay weakened and dazed on the grass in front of the marquee which was shattered beyond repair. Between soft groans, she mumbled, "I never ever wasbad. I never ever cried." Sniffling, she mumbled in child-like innocence, "Whywon'tGod . . . Why won't He giveme a miracle?"

As the paramedics lifted her onto the gurney and rolled her into the ambulance, Sam heard her mother's voice echo in her addled brain. It was the same sinister voice her mother used each time Sam asked why her father sodomized her. Her mother's glacially detached answer was always the same. "He's a man."

Heavily sedated, Sam floated in and out of consciousness as the nurse adjusted the instruments attached to her. At the nurse's station, one nurse asked the other, "Who's the *Jen* 211 keeps asking for?"

"I'm not sure," the other nurse answered. "All she's been mumbling since they brought her in is, 'Jen will help me.'"

Placing several charts in the file cabinet, the nurse said, "Maybe we'll get lucky if we scan her cell."

The nurse's hunch proved fruitful. Within seconds, she tapped Jenna Rossi Gaone's number, and the phone rang.

Steve yelled up the stairs, "Hey diva, we need to be at the restaurant by five, and your phone's ringing."

"Get it while I grab my purse."

Steve said, "Hello."

"May I speak with Jenna Gaone, please?"

Puzzled by the woman's formal tone, Steve inquired, "May I ask who's calling?"

"My name is Erin Rich. I'm a psychiatric nurse at Monroeville Hospital."

His chin dropped to his chest.

Jenna started down the stairs and asked, "What's wrong?"

Handing her the phone, he mouthed, "Samantha Kind."

"Sam, I can't talk right now, I'm—"

"Jenna Gaone?"

Confused, she shot Steve a puzzled look and said to the voice, "I'm sorry; I thought I was talking to my friend, Samantha."

Steve pointed to his watch.

Jenna shrugged.

"Samantha Kind was admitted to Monroeville Psychiatric Center this afternoon, but we don't have a next of kin or any insurance information. She's been repeating your name. Would you be able to furnish the name of a family member we can contact?"

"Sam has no family, but I'm her friend who usually helps her manage situations like this."

"She can use a good friend right now. Would you be willing to meet with her doctor on staff so we can work from a history?"

"Of course. I can be there by late morning."

"We'll be expecting you then."

Steve plopped in a chair, eyed Jenna, and asked, "What now?"

Masking her fear, she casually fastened her earring and said, "Sam's on a psych ward. They need info on her, and she needs help making medical decisions."

He tossed his keys on the table. "My client, who I'm standing up as we speak, expects to be on a boat with us tomorrow morning. Did it occur to you that while your nutty friend usurps your time, I need your support with clients like him to maintain a thriving business?"

Faking nonchalance, she said, "Stop insulting my friend, and let's go entertain yours. Just tell him the truth. Most people with a heart understand that a person with emotional problems needs support."

Put off by her implication, he said, "Just because I don't jump through hoops every time the Queen of Quack calls, doesn't mean I'm heartless." Softening, he took a deep breath, straightened his tie, and picked up the keys. "How bad is she?"

Jenna stopped short of the door. Unable to hold back blistering tears, she swung around and cried, "Why can't I stop her pain?" Through clenched teeth, she said, "Nothing I do or say ever stops her pain."

Pulling her close, Steve felt her body quake with sobs.

"Jenna, if everything Sam says is true, you stop the pain each time you tell her you love her, each time you insist she's a good person. God only knows how many times she would have killed herself or someone else had you not been attentive to her. You pick up the phone every blessed time she calls."

Dabbing her eyes with a tissue, she asked, "What am I supposed to do? She's been waiting a lifetime for someone to put her at the top of the list to be loved. I can't stand the thought of them pumping her with medication, turning her into a zombie. She needs life around her to be spotless; she needs people to listen to her ramble. She needs—"

"Stop it, Jen. She's finally where she needs to be. For a few days, anyway."

Jenna offered a weak nod, dabbed her nose, and said, "Let's go before you lose your client."

Resigned, he said, "We can make dinner tonight, but we'll tell them Sam needs us for the next few days."

Mildly surprised, she asked, "You're jeopardizing business for Sam?"

Palming the back of her neck, he pulled her toward him, and said, "For you. Stop talking and let's go."

Between ordering the filet mignon and sipping on the Cabernet Sauvignon, Steve and Jenna learned that their client had a niece suffering from a bipolar disorder. She was under the care of a doctor referred to their family by Dr. Mark Packard.

"Although Packard mainly works with veterans, he's been known to extend himself to patients with stress disorders outside the military realm," the client told them.

"I grew up with Mark Packard," Jenna said, intentionally avoiding discussion of the accident that killed her brother, Josh.

The client's wife widened her eyes. "That's a stroke of luck. My sister-in-law tells me he's a wonderful man. You can count on him to offer sound advice." She threw her husband a knowing look.

"He's not one to make the situation worse, like several questionable psychiatrists we've encountered."

As the evening ended, Steve thanked his client again for understanding, and he promised to have his secretary reschedule a meeting at the earliest date.

Back home, Steve loosened his tie, sat on the couch, and said, "Sometimes I feel like we're the only sane people on the planet." After checking his messages, he tossed his phone aside, and asked, "When do you want to contact Packard?"

"Do you think he'll want to help Sam?"

Massaging his temples, he said, "He's not gonna say *no* to you."

"Let's listen to what the doctor in Monroeville has to say. I'll call Mark from there."

Jenna curled up next to Steve and laid her head on his chest. Wondering aloud, she asked, "Why does life heap difficulties on some people, and others sail by without a care?"

"Don't go down that road, Jen. The world's strewn with angry, resentful people who waste time trying to figure out why bad things happen to good people." He let out a sarcastic laugh. "None of us are as good as we'd like to think we are. We're all prodigals."

"You have to admit; some people carry more burdens for longer periods than others."

"I won't deny some people have an easier time surviving, but the more fortunate people by and large seem to answer the call to lend help and hope to the weary." Massaging her back, he said, "Your problem is you've been trying to change the world for Sam, but the world doesn't change for anyone." He nudged her and said, "Let's get some rest. Something tells me we're in for a rocky ride."

Jenna and Steve arrived at the hospital by ten in the morning. He waited in the lounge as the nurse escorted Jenna to Sam's room. Jenna surveyed the cubicle, stopping for a moment to stare at another patient singing *Rain, Rain Go Away*. Blinking hard, she swung her eyes to

Sam, who was softly groaning. Gently holding Sam's bandaged hand, she said, "I'm here. We'll do this together."

Fearing severe discipline for her violent actions, Sam forced herself to hold back a flood of tears. A soft whine escaped her lips before she whispered, "Tell them I'll be good. I promise." Her lower lip quivered when she said, "I'llbegood."

"No one's gonna hurt you, Sam. The medicine's calming you. I'm here. I'll stay as long as you need me."

"Take me home," she whispered. "I wanna go home."

Gently brushing Sam's hair out of her face, Jenna told her, "This time I found one of the best doctors in the country to help us. His name's Mark Packard."

Hanging on to Jenna's every word, Sam shook her head in confusion. She whimpered, "No, not him. He killed Josh." Bursting into tears, she said, "I should've died, not little Josh. We'd all be happy, and . . . and I need a drink, Jen, justalittledrink to calm . . ." Her voice trailed off.

"Don't think like that, Sam. You're gonna live and be happy, and we'll be friends forever."

"Okay, okay, okay," she whispered trying to assure herself as fear mixed with futility.

Jenna stood back as the nurse pulled the white curtain around Sam's bed to check her vital signs.

Sam cried out, "Jenna! Don't go!"

Jenna pulled a chair closer to the bed and said, "I'm right here, Sam. I'll sit right here while you rest."

"I love you, Jen." Large tears welled in her eyes bulging with fear. "You're the only one," she whispered breathlessly, "who comes."

Jenna handed Sam a tissue and wrapped her arms around her. "I love you, too, Sam." She planted a soft kiss on her forehead. "I'll talk to the doctor, but this time you have to cooperate."

Her eyelids weighed heavy from the medication, but before she slipped into a deep sleep, she mumbled, "I promise to . . . I promise."

Gulping their lunches, Steve and Jenna raced through mid-day traffic to make a two o'clock appointment with Sam's assigned doctor at the psychiatric hospital. After a lengthy discussion, Jenna stood to leave.

She turned and said, "We want to contact Dr. Mark Packard from The Art of Healing Institute and ask him to render an opinion."

The doctor's eyes widened. "Packard's hardly accessible to the public. His research and practice focus more on combat vets suffering PTSD. I don't know how much interest he'll have in a child abuse case."

"My wife knows him," Steve said.

The doctor raised his brows. "I'd be fascinated to hear what he has to say."

"We'll contact Dr. Packard from the hotel. I'll be back this evening to stay with Sam until she rests for the night." With a plea in her voice, Jenna said, "Reassure Sam, doctor. Make her know that you, we all care about her."

Lounging in their hotel room, Jenna told Steve, "I imagine Packard's gone for the day."

"That man's not a nine-to-five guy. Even if he's away from his office," Steve countered, "he'll check his messages. As soon as he hears the name *Rossi*, he won't be able to dial fast enough."

"What makes you so sure?" she asked, resting her head on two stacked pillows.

Crawling on the bed and snuggling close to her, he said, "Because if anyone's indebted to the Rossis, Mark Packard is."

"Stop saying that, Stephen." Holding her phone up, she asked, "Do you think I should call now?"

Nodding, he told her, "It will give him time to schedule a meeting in the next few days."

"It takes us a month to schedule a car inspection, and you think Mark's going to say, 'Y'all come down to one of the busiest hospitals in the country right this minute, ya hear?'"

Drawing her into his arms, he said, "You underestimate the power of guilt."

She wiggled free saying, "You're groping the queen of guilt." She dialed Mark Packard's number. As the phone rang, she added, "The last thing I want is to capitalize on his guilt."

He pointed at her and said, "That man will feel guilty 'til the day he dies."

After the fourth ring, an enthusiastic secretary answered asking, "The Art of Healing Institute, how may I help you?"

"Hi, my name is Jenna Rossi Gaone. I grew up with Dr. Packard, and I'm in an emergency where I can sure use his expert advice. Will you please pass my name on to him? I would appreciate his input at his convenience."

"Please hold, Ms. Gaone."

Several seconds passed before Mark Packard's voice interrupted Beethoven's *Sixth Symphony (The Pastoral)* playing while she waited. He said her name with unmistakable surprise.

"Jenna?"

"I'm so sorry for bothering you, but I don't have anywhere else to turn."

Shaking off mild shock, Dr. Packard sat in his leather swivel chair and nervously strung several sentences together in rapid succession. "I'm glad you called. Of course, I'll help you. I read about the hostage crisis and your marriage to Steve Gaone. I hear only good things about him. Where are you?"

"Steve and I are staying at the West Wind Bed and Breakfast in Monroeville." Motioning a thumbs up to Steve, she added, "We've been following your success as well, Dr. Packard."

His voice soft and low, he said, "Please, Jenna, call me Mark." After a short pause, he asked, "How can I help you?"

"Do you remember Samantha Kind? She lived down the street from me when we were kids."

"I never met her, but I remember hearing talk about the double murder of her parents for weeks after it happened."

"Sam was eighteen when she shot her father after he killed her mother and threatened to kill her. That was after her parents physically and sexually abused her from the time she was an infant. She's been attached to a questionable psychiatrist who seems to be making Sam's situation worse, but the immediate concern is just yesterday she lost control of herself. She vandalized a church marquee because she didn't get a miracle from God. Until now, she's been a functioning alcoholic, but yesterday her irrational behavior landed her on the Monroeville psych ward. She's been traumatized all her life; she's obsessive about cleanliness, and she has major trust issues, especially with men. If all that isn't bad enough, she has no family, no support system, and I've been her only real friend for the past ten years." Clearing her throat, she asked, "Does anything in this madness sound like something you can help redirect, help her find a path to some small measure of peace in her tormented life?"

Before he could answer, Jenna pleaded Sam's case by adding, "She's a good person, Mark. Some of our lives get derailed, but we're able to get back on track because people loved us and guided us. She's suffered all her life, and everyone's always brushing her aside, and I don't know what else . . . I'm running out of . . ." Her throat constricted before letting out several soft, nervous sobs.

Steve handed her a tissue and whispered, "You're doing great."

She dabbed her eyes, cleared her throat, and said, "I'm sorry. I'm rambling like a lunatic myself."

"No, no, Jenna. Don't ever apologize for loving someone enough to share his or her pain. Sometimes it's just as difficult for family members to watch loved ones sink into a dark place. The patient can't get out, and loved ones can't get in."

"I know you work with vets suffering from PTSD, but I believe Sam's abuse left her traumatized beyond even a soldier's torment."

"Right now, all the residents at my facility are vets, but you're spot-on about trauma disorders. The patients harbor toxic memories, demons from an array of experiences. Severe trauma resulting in stress disorders locks the individual in a hell that robs him of his spirit and will. We do everything we can to help soothe, redirect, and in some cases, heal the wounds. The sooner we get patients to interact with others who've experienced the same trauma under the same circumstances, the better results we have. From a realistic standpoint, undoing thirty-three years of trauma beginning in the formative years will be difficult, but maybe we can reach an acceptable level of management. My clinic's a couple of hours away from Monroeville. If you're able to meet with me day after tomorrow, it will give me time to study her folder." More excited, he said, "I'd love to give you a tour of the place. You can decide if The Institute's where she can find some level of comfort and aid. Have Samantha's doctor fax her records. We'll go from there."

Mildly shocked at his immediate response to her request, Jenna said, "I don't expect you to disrupt your routine for—"

He was quick to say, "I want to . . . I need to do this, Jenna. I've wanted to talk with you and your parents for years, but I never had the . . ." He cleared his throat. "Even if I don't work with your friend directly, I'll recommend someone who will offer her the help she needs. Please, let me do this for you."

Wide-eyed, Jenna turned to Steve, and asked, "Day after tomorrow?"

Steve winked and mouthed, "Called it."

"I'll notify Sam's doctor tonight, and we'll see you soon."

She jumped on the bed and said, "He just rearranged his full day to accommodate us."

Playfully trying to disrobe her, Steve said, "That guy's been waiting his whole career to help a Rossi."

She gently slapped his hand, stood and straightened out her blouse. "I promised Sam I'd tuck her in, and we have to talk to the nurse to make sure they fax Sam's records to Mark."

He stood, crossed his arms over his chest, and said with a mock pout, "You're forgetting that I've rearranged a couple of days of my life for you. I'm not budging until you promise to tuck me in when we get back."

She sauntered into his arms and said, "I'm aware of what you do for me. Every time life sucker punches me, you pull me into these big, muscular arms and make the pain bearable." Tapping his nose, she told him, "I'll tuck you in on one condition, cowboy. You have to make love to me nice and slow so that I—"

Grabbing her tighter, he kissed her long on the lips. "You drive the hardest bargains, Mrs. Gaone."

Sam sat silent in her bed fighting the urge to throw a pitcher of water at her roommate singing *Rain, Rain Go Away*, for what seemed like the millionth time in a light-year of torture. When Jenna walked into the room, Sam's eyes swung to her.

"Puhleeze! Can't you get me out of this filthy place?" She clutched the sides of her head and pressed hard over her ears. "If I hear that song from that crazy loon one more time I'll," she glared at her fellow psych patient, "rip her vocal chords out." Covering her face with her hands, she whispered, "I need a drink sooo bad. The food tastes like meat someone left on the counter for three days, and they make me take showers in that," she said, pointing to the bathroom facility. "You can smell the stench from across the room." Crossing her arms over her chest, she squeezed tightly and said with defiance, "And tell them not to touch . . . I'm not letting any one of them eeever touch me." In a child-like voice she pleaded, "I wanna go home."

"We're all trying to help you, Sam. Going back home right now will put you at square one. Give Mark Packard a chance to come up with a plan to make you well."

Sam slammed her head back hard on her pillow as her angry tear-rimmed eyes glared at Jenna. She whispered through clenched teeth, "All's I wanted was a miracle from God. Is that too much to ask?" More child-like, she said, "All's I wanted was for them to love me. All's I wanted . . . Who cares anyway?" Fighting back tears, Sam asked, "Why's everyone doing this to me? I'll pay for the damn lying marquee. Why'd that church put up a sign that lied? I'm sooo sick of liars."

A nurse walked into the room, filled Sam's glass with fresh water, and said, "I have something that'll calm you, sweetie."

Sam put the pill in her mouth and let the nurse watch her swallow. She rested her head on the pillow and began to mumble under her breath, "Stopspying. Can't get away from spies."

As the medication coursed through Sam's system, she whispered in a barely audible voice, "Holdme, Jen. Don't let them hurt . . . . . . I'magoodgirl." Her eyes rolled back as she dropped into oblivion.

Jenna brushed strands of hair away from Sam's cheeks, planted a soft kiss on her forehead, and whispered, "This time you'll get well."

The receptionist at Dr. Mark Packard's The Art of Healing Institute offered Jenna and Steve coffee while they waited in his office. Already a half hour late, Dr. Packard sprinted across campus, burst through the door, and extended his hand. Out of breath, he said, "Sorry for the delay. One of the residents was in a rare talkative mood, and I never dissuade dialogue."

Jenna smiled at the receptionist and said, "This kind lady kept us comfortable."

Tall, square-faced, and soft spoken, Mark Packard palmed Sam's folder lying on his desk and said, "I'd like more time to study the details." He held up the folder. "Samantha Kind's story is gritty." Easing back in his leather chair, he asked in amazement, "Are you really her only support?"

With a slight shrug, Jenna said, "It's been that way ever since she moved our senior year in high school and her father and mother died."

"It's challenging to vault over an isolated, traumatic war event, but this? I've never encountered an individual who's lived, let alone survived, a lifetime of trauma." Grabbing a notepad, he told Jenna and Steve, "I've listed several facilities suited for her needs. I'll oversee her treatment, but because of the nature of the sexual abuse, I recommend a female doctor."

Steve eyed Mark before asking, "May I be frank?"

"I'd appreciate that."

"Is your decision to work with Sam based on professional belief that there's real hope for her, or are you simply extending a kindness to the Rossis?"

Jenna swung her disapproving eyes to Steve.

Mark said, "Fair question." Eyeing Jenna, he said, "Both. I tackle each case with a large dose of hope, but from what I know of Samantha's experiences, the odds are stacked against her." He tapped his pen several times before explaining, "Think of it in terms of animals in their natural habitat. If a bird is born and raised in a cage, chances are it'll fear flying out of that cage even when you free it to fly. The same phenomenon happens with animals raised in a zoo. Many would fail miserably at foraging for food and protecting themselves against predators in uncontrolled nature." His sympathetic eyes canvassed Jenna when he told her, "Sam may understand love intellectually, but she may lack the ability to express love emotionally. Sporadic periods of friendship and love, especially in the formative years, generally are insufficient to build a foundation upon which one can sustain a journey to wellness." He asked Jenna point blank, "You know her best. Has she gotten better over the years or worse?"

Steve shot Jenna a dubious look.

"I don't know," she said, her voice doubtful. "She never talked about the abuse in grade school, but since the day she killed her father, she talks of little else. She's like a needle trapped in a deep scratch on a vinyl record. I nudge her onto other topics, and she's fine for a brief time. Then her mind slips back into the groove where she stays stuck until I force her to . . . I'm not sure. I don't know if . . ." Her voice, confused and uncertain, trailed off.

His knowing eyes rested on her. "I have no delusions about what will and will not work here. While your commitment to her is evident and admirable, we need to accept the fact that Samantha may be incapable of achieving an acceptable level of normalcy. She may act rational at times, but think of a child's mind developing in the same way a physical body develops. If a child spends a lifetime confined in a small box, he emerges with deformed bones and atrophied muscles. The best physical therapy in the world will only improve those muscles and bones to a certain point. The same concept applies to cognitive and emotional growth. Samantha's exceptionally bright, but the years of abuse more than likely caused some permanent damage to her emotional capacity." He removed his glasses and tucked them in his shirt pocket. "No matter how much you want a better life for her, Jenna, she needs to want it more, and she needs to be able at some level to achieve it on her own." Shaking his head, he tapped Samantha's folder with his index finger. "If it's any consolation, know unequivocally, your friendship throughout the years carried her farther than her folder indicates she would have gotten otherwise."

Steve gently squeezed Jenna's hand and told Mark, "I'm not sure those records adequately describe some of the strengths Sam has going for her."

"Undocumented factors have a lot to do with a patient's progress, so what positives do you believe may help?"

Steve looked at Jenna and said, "You always talk about how Sam rarely missed a day of school. How Josh got a black eye fighting those kids teasing her. Your mother cooked her angel hair pasta almost every Sunday, and Josh sneaked it to her on occasion." Swinging his eyes to Mark, he said, "Surely the constant of Jenna always answering the phone combined with those other kindnesses have to register in some positive way."

He lowered his eyes at the mention of Josh's name, but quickly made eye contact with Steve, and said, "No doubt. The positive interaction at school's a big plus, too." He turned his eyes to Jenna and said, "Let's pray that the seeds of hope and love your family planted in her bear enough strength and hope for her to fight."

Sitting on the edge of his desk, his sympathetic eyes washed over Jenna. "The last concern I have is how you'll react if this experiment ends badly."

Letting out a sarcastic laugh, she said, "The worst that can happen is I'll have to listen to her horror stories for the rest of my life."

Furrowing his brow, he said, "I'm afraid that's not the worst." He admitted, "Despite my objections, several patients over the years have released themselves from my facility sooner than recommended, convinced they were able to manage their demons without medication and therapy. Suicide proved more painless. With Sam, we also can't rule out the capacity to harm others."

Wide eyed, she asked, "Are you referring to that maverick cop's theory about the double murder?"

"When I Googled articles on the murder, the discrepancies concern me, but I don't know enough to offer an informed legal opinion. I do know that when a traumatized patient has the capacity to lose touch with reality, the patient and those around the patient may be in danger."

Comforting Jenna, Steve said, "He's discussing considerations."

Shoulders slumped, a soft pout formed on her lips. "Maybe we shouldn't push her."

Steve swung his eyes to Mark.

Mark tilted his head and said, "My intuition tells me Samantha's at a crossroads. You wouldn't be sitting in my office if you didn't share that feeling. She won't be able to function much longer without inflicting damage on herself and others if she hasn't already." Sitting back in his chair, he sized Jenna up, and said, "If Samantha played a more prominent role in the murders of her parents, we could be dealing with a homicidal sociopath who's intelligent enough to play the system, yet emotionally deficient enough to minimize her harmful behavior. I'd feel more comfortable studying her case more before I reject the detective's assertion that Sam manipulated evidence at the crime scene." As an aside, Mark said, "I read an account where the detective claims he receives threatening notes from Samantha Kind, but he can't prove it."

Steve swung his eyes to Jenna. "How about all the times she threatens to harm you and me?"

"It's a rumor, Steve." Her eyes on Mark, she said, "How can she whine like a child one minute and be a criminal mastermind the next?"

Tapping his pen on the desk, Mark told her, "The dichotomy in personalities can exist. Her underdeveloped childish emotions may drive her negative behavior, while her more developed intellect allows her to manipulate others and rationalize her injurious behavior. All I'm saying is we need to keep an open mind." He picked up Sam's medical folder and said, "The preliminary review indicates she's badly broken, as emotionally damaged as I've seen in all my years of practice. I wouldn't be surprised if she suffers a personality disorder. Emotionally damaged people generally craft veneers to fit into society. Mass murderer, Eileen Wuornos from the famed movie *Monster* is an extreme example."

Jenna pulled back. "They executed that woman."

"That's how bad situations like this can get," Mark told her. "While Sam seems to share similar qualities, all we can do is give it our best shot and hope she lacks the sociopathic traits and cooperates with treatment. Some level of normality, if it's to come at all, won't be quick; it won't be easy, and it will take years of monitoring to keep Sam and everyone around her safe."

As Steve and Jenna stood to leave, Mark fidgeted. In an awkward attempt to keep Jenna in the office longer, he asked, "How are your parents?"

Steve pointed to the door. "I'll grab some coffee in the cafeteria. Catch up with me when you're done here."

Jenna sat and said, "My mom and dad are well. They're proud of what you've done with your life."

His eyes glistened. "Not a day goes by that I don't think about," his voice cracked, "Josh." He ran his hand through his hair, held it for a second, and said, "That day in court, after your dad petitioned the judge for leniency, I had every intention of being dead by morning."

Jenna gasped.

Tapping his temple with his index finger, he said, "I couldn't get it out of my mind. Josh was dead because of me. Those weeks before the hearing, every time I looked at my own brother . . ." He shook his head. "I stopped talking to him; I couldn't touch him."

Jenna's eyes blurred. "My parents would be heartbroken if they knew Josh was the reason for so much unhappiness."

"I know," he whispered. "Your father visited my house that night after the hearing and asked my parents if he could talk with me." He smiled saying, "When I heard his voice in the foyer, I thought for sure he changed his mind and decided to grab me by my scrawny throat and strangle me to death with his bare hands." He tapped his pen on the desk and said with wonder, "But he didn't." Looking down for a second to gain composure, his eyes raised and locked with hers. "Your father draped his arm over my shoulders and told me, 'I never met a man with strength of character who didn't have some sad stories to tell, some regrets.' He tousled my hair, like he really cared about me." Mark's eyes looked at her, but his senses relived the scene a lifetime ago. "Not a day goes by that I don't hear your dad's voice saying, 'Rosie and I are counting on you to live a good life, Mark, not only for yourself, but for our Josh.'" Mark blinked back tears. "Your dad taught me that people are able to make it through any kind of trauma when someone or something gives them a reason to bear the pain."

Mark stood and opened his arms to Jenna.

She gave him a long, tight hug and said, "Look at this place! If all that you do here isn't scoring a victory for humanity, I don't know what does." Pointing at him, she warned with a tease, "Next time you see your brother, promise me you'll grab him in a bear hug. If he pushes you away, grab him tighter."

He let out a sigh, palmed his chest, and said, "I'm overwhelmed that you trust me with the care of someone you love. I'll do everything in my power to make this work."

Admiring the campus facilities that promised peace to so many who moved through life in torment, Jenna wended her way to the cafeteria. A gentle breeze swirled around her, playing with her hair, her cheeks, her heart. She stopped, drew in a light breath, and whispered to her brother's loving spirit, "I love you back."

Chapter Twenty-Three

AFTER FULFILLING SEVERAL MONTHS OF PERSONAL AND professional obligations, Jenna petitioned for an overdue sabbatical from her teaching position, and Steve scheduled time off from his business. Their ten-day trip to Rome provided the first quality, private time they enjoyed together since their honeymoon. On the next to the last day of their getaway, Steve slid the curtain to one side and interrupted Jenna's shower. She squealed with delight as he picked her up and clumsily dropped her on the bed.

"You're clean enough *Il mio cuore e l'anima.*"

"Be patient *dio dell' amore,*" she seductively scolded, wiping the water from her face with her hands. "I'm giving my *god of love* a clean body to go along with a *clean heart and soul.* Besides, we have dinner reservations in an hour."

"Forget the restaurant. I'll feast on you," he said, nibbling her neck.

Staring into his eager eyes, she massaged his back as he lay on top of her. "Man-up, cowboy. You're escorting me to an elegant restaurant, and I'm going to stuff myself with delicacies."

He whispered breathlessly, "I'm all for stuffing you with delicacies, my love."

"I'm savoring you for dessert," she teased, coaxing him to dress for dinner.

They arrived on schedule at the *Restorante L'Archeologia* where myriad of wines lined the deep red walls. Open fires exuded romance and charm. The day being warmer than usual, they opted for outdoor seating in the refreshing shade of the centuries-old gardens where pale bluish clusters of lilac flowers climbed the walls and hung from pergolas. Feeling fortunate to catch an evening when jazz musicians set the night to music, they leisurely dined on tasty Italian cuisines that complemented the aesthetic beauty surrounding them. After dinner, they slipped back in time as they first toured the well-stocked wine cellar and then strolled the Appian Road where ancient monuments echoed Roman past.

The next morning, sightseeing at the Vatican, Jenna traded reverence for mild mockery as she wound her way up the sloping five hundred, fifty-one steps of the Cupola. Steve lagged close behind, not quite sure what to expect when he reached the top of the narrowing spiral stairway.

"Keep moving, Stephen," she teased. "If you can't fit though the opening, you'll have to turn around and go back down."

Dumbfounded, he looked up at Jenna and asked, "Do you really believe after climbing five hundred stairs, the people following me will graciously consent to an about face?" He shooed her away saying, "To the top, *bella*, before they trample me to death."

"Relax, sweetie. If a chubby pope like John XXIII made it through this opening, so can you."

"Hey, Jen, I'll wager my muscular torso that John XXIII opted for the elevator."

Huffing and puffing, a man following Steve let out a laugh. "Hey muscle man, if there's an elevator, why're we all on these steps inviting heart attacks?"

Steve glanced over his shoulder. "Does the word *beneficiary* mean anything to you?"

The man's wife climbing directly behind him said, "It would be more lucrative for us to kill you at home. Transporting a body from Rome to JFK is expensive, between five to eight thousand dollars." Letting out a short laugh, she said, "Then again, if we cremate you here, they'll only charge us about a thousand dollars. We can even carry your ashes on the plane and stuff you in the overhead compartment."

Steve looked over the man's head and shot the woman a wry grin. He stared at the man, narrowed his eyes, and teased, "I'd be concerned about your wife's inordinate knowledge of transporting dead bodies if I were you."

Their shared laughter, though brief, gave them a needed break from the taxing climb. Crawling up the last several steps, he contorted his body, which enabled him to slip through the opening with more ease than he anticipated. Standing atop the observation deck, they admired the panoramic view of Rome.

Pointing across the city, he said, "See, way out there; that's the Pantheon."

"That's irony for ya," Jenna quipped. "We're standing on top of St. Peter's Basilica, God's seat on earth, and directly across from it," she pointed to the Pantheon, "is the structure that housed all the pagan gods throughout the centuries."

He pulled her close. "You're so much smarter than your class standing."

Gently kissing his cheek, she said, "Life's always presenting dualities of good and evil. I wonder if—"

Her phone rang.

Before she could tell Steve who it was, he said, "Please, don't ruin this magnificent moment for me." He turned, held the binoculars to his eyes and surveyed Rome while Jenna consoled Sam.

Sam's voice rose above the *glug, glug, glug* of a drink she was pouring. "Puhleeze don't be mad, Jen. I just couldn't take those people in that prison any more. The bathrooms were so filthy."

"Where are you?" Her heart sinking at the thought of Sam's relapse after months of intensive therapy, she said, "'Those people' are trying to help you get your life together. You need to go back. Don't give them a reason to cut you from the program."

Sam snapped saying, "That's not gonna happen. I'm never goin' back. They can't tell me . . . You can't tell me what to do. I was bossed around all my life. I'm capable of making my own decisions, thank you."

"Mark Packard pulled all kinds of strings to get you the help you need. You'll never find a more qualified doctor. Give him a few more months."

Dizzying and more incoherent as the conversation dragged on, Sam said, "He'sakiller. Killed lil'Josh, and youthink . . . Youthink I'm the one," she burped, "who'scrazy? Lock him up, not me." Glass clinked against the phone as she swallowed hard. "He's like everyotherman. Women do all the grunge work while he, he, he collects all the goodies." After several moments of silence interrupted by a hiccup, she said, "And I don't 'preciate people always askin' mequestions. They ask 'bout the day my parents died. They wannablame *me*." After a short pause, she gained more lucidity and said, "You always tell me to silence the ghosts. How? Tell me how. Help me git these people ta stop talkin' 'bout something I wanna forget." She muttered under her breath, "MarkPackard's a murderer, not me."

"Mark's the best there is, Sam. He wants to help you—"

Making nonsensical noises to drown Jenna's voice, Sam sang, "Na na, na na, na na . . . Not gonnahappen. Nevergonnahappen because . . ." She stopped short and blurted out, "Where are you, anyway, Jenna? Why'd you stick me in that hell-hole and never visit me?"

"You signed the admissions form, Sam. They suggested I give you time to adjust. Mark talks to your doctor on a regular basis, and the doctor updates me. It's the best help a person can find for trauma. Trust me, Sam."

Laughing sarcastically, she said, "You stick me with a murderer, and I haven't seen or heard from yer sorry ass in weeks, and you want me to trust . . . Where are you?" she yelled. "I drove all the way ta yer house. Stopped at yer mother's. No one's home anywhere. Where's everyone, Jenna? It's like I've crossed over in to the damn *Twilight Zone*!" she screamed, causing Jenna to hold the phone away from her ear.

Pressing the tips of her fingers hard on her eyelids, Jenna's curt voice said, "We'll be home tomorrow evening. I'll smooth the situation over with Mark Packard."

"Are you deaf? I'm never goin' back. I'm livin'the way I want ta live, so stay . . . Just stay where you are. Let that tog . . . I mean hog . . . screw you 'til you can't remember who or what you ever were. Soon you won't . . . You won't recognize yourself. That's what men do to us, Jenna. You think you're so special?"

Jenna tried to reason with Sam before silence signaled she wasn't there.

Frustrated, Jenna shoved her phone in her purse, looked up, and caught Steve's eyes.

"Sam dropped out of—"

He held up his hand.

Studying Rome for several moments, he turned to Jenna, and said, "Time to cut her loose."

Instead of mounting her usual defense of Sam, Jenna zeroed in on the Pantheon. Wondering aloud, she said, "It's amazing how society admires and protects cold, empty monuments from abuse and deterioration, but we abandon with ease and discard abused and deteriorating human beings."

Dropping his head, he rested his chin on his chest for several seconds before looking up and saying, "I'm not suggesting that you discard her. I asked you to let her go. If she can't or won't help us help her, coddling her only delays the painful inevitable."

"What's the inevitable, Steve? Living a cold, empty life without a single friend? Drinking herself to death?"

He pulled her close. "You need to stop acting like her tortured life is somehow your fault."

"I have everything. What does she have? Me!"

His loving eyes canvassed her face. Teasing, he said, "While we're here, let's mark off where they should place Saint Jenna the Martyr's statue."

Her eyes watered when she asked, "Why didn't my mother force Child Protection Services to help Sam? The adults knew what was happening to her."

Deadpanned, he said, "You've been listening to Sam for so long, she's brainwashed you into thinking distorted thoughts like her. Your mother opened her house and heart to that girl. Your whole family loved her." Drawing Jenna back into his arms, he said, "Mark warned us that even after all the trying, sometimes we can't make it better. Sometimes we lose."

Although the pain of Sam's relapse threatened to hijack Jenna's joy at visiting the Vatican museum, Steve's non-stop itinerary diverted her attention to the memorable beauty surrounding them at every turn. As the sun faded into the horizon, they strolled the evening along the Piazza Navona with its beautiful fountains and Baroque architecture. They shared a drink and raised a toast to love.

Wiggling and squirming at the sight of Jenna and Steve for the first time in ten days, Noce broke loose from Clare's car and bound up the driveway.

With equal enthusiasm, Jenna grabbed the dog, traded kisses, and sang, "Noce Baby! Did you miss your mommy?"

Noce licked Jenna's cheeks and caught the corner of her mouth several times prompting Steve to warn, "Don't come near me until you've bathed away that doggie saliva dripping from your beautiful face."

Steve carried the last piece of luggage up the stairs while Jenna and Clare watched Noce tear back and forth through the yard, ecstatic to romp on her own turf.

"So, what's the most beautiful sight in Italy?" Clare asked.

"Just one?" Jenna countered.

"Did you climb the Cupola?"

"Sure did! Everyone behind Steve crowned him the Cupola King for managing to slip through the opening."

Clare handed Noce's leash to Jenna and said, "I thought the dog would cause more grief, but the sweetheart was an ad for model pet behavior. Makes me want to adopt a puppy from the pound, but Tony enjoys his freedom." She kissed Jenna on the cheek and said, "You feed the puppy, and I'll go feed your father-in-law. Call if you need us."

Jenna calmed the dog before climbing the stairs to help Steve unpack. Catching him off guard, he jumped up from the desk and subtly shoved a small object into his pants pocket.

"What're you writing?"

"A *to do* list," he lied.

Skeptical, she asked, "Why so skittish?" Moving closer, she grabbed his belt with a tease, and asked, "What's in your pocket, cowboy?"

Fending her off, he said, "By the time you brush that doggie breath out of your mouth, I'll be done here."

She placed her hands on her hips and argued, "Like Noce kissing me two times smells worse than my eating a five-pound catfish before you suck my face down your throat."

He grabbed her in a bear hug and said, "That's because you're one tasty Italian lady." He playfully nudged her toward the bed and added, "You're hot and spicy, and—"

As he tumbled on top of her, she tapped his nose, and said, "Just a second ago my doggie breath repelled you. Now, I'm tasty?"

"Your body hygiene is within the boundaries of safe sex," he teased, grabbing her lips with his mouth.

"Convincing me I'm clean enough to make love with you won't get you lucky, cowboy." Rolling him to the side, she stood, and tugged at his jeans. "Show me what you have stashed in those pants."

Bare chested and tight jeans, he eyed her seductively, and coaxed, "Dig in and get it, baby. It's all yours."

Several exaggerated lusty groans escaped him as she thrust her hand down deep into his pocket, executing a longer and rougher than necessary search. After retrieving a necklace, she was giddy crawling back onto the bed.

Her finger gently skimmed the surface of the diamond teardrop. "Can I wear it now?" she asked with excitement.

"Yes, you may," he corrected her.

Ignoring his condescension, she held the ends together and let him clasp it. He gently rolled on top of her and said, "Several weeks before we landed, I called the most exquisite jeweler in Rome and asked if he would design it for me."

"So, that explains why I waited forty-five minutes in the hotel garden wondering where you were Monday evening," she said, fondling the teardrop.

His lips brushed hers as he said, "I appreciated your understanding."

She let out a laugh and said, "When the most gorgeous guy on earth escorts you to Italy, you don't pick a fight." More seriously, she asked, "Why a teardrop?"

He kissed one eye and then the other. "These beautiful eyes shed tears for so many people. No matter how many times life knocks you down, you get back up and fight, not just for yourself, but for everyone you care about."

Massaging her chest, he told her, "Your tears overflow into my heart, making it stretch wider than the sky."

He pressed his body down on hers and whispered, "Procreate with me."

Her hands glided up and down his muscular back as she asked in a sultry voice, "Did I ever tell you about the first time I dreamed of procreating with you?"

"You've mentioned babies from time to time."

"Remember when you caught me daydreaming that first evening we were together at The Renaissance Inn?"

"Vaguely." Touching his temple, he said, "The one memory that obscures all others from that night is how I made you cry."

Her eyes swept over his face. Gently tracing his lips with her fingertips, she said, "I thought the Vatican was the most magnificent place I'd ever been, but I was wrong. Right here," she said, planting a kiss on his forehead; "here," she whispered, kissing his chest. Wrapping her arms around his neck, she told him, "Your head and heart are the most beautiful places I've ever been, and I want to stay there forever."

"Play me," he begged.

She whispered obligingly, "Jazz? Classic? Rock?"

His eager eyes swept over her with anticipation. "Let's do a medley."

Her gentle strokes began to draw from him sweet passionate melodies that set their hearts to music well into the night.

Chapter Twenty-Four

HOLDING UP A CAN OF BEER, PHIL CALLED OUT, "HAPPY birthday, Michael! Two more years and you'll be legal."

Mike pushed the bottle away and said, "Now, that's what entrapment's all about."

Phil draped his arm over Mike's shoulder and asked, "Any hot chicks chasing you?"

"Next Friday I'm hooking up with a medical student from C. A. Hooker College, a small school about a half hour away from campus."

A broad smile flashed across Phil's face. "See a hooker?" He swung his eyes to his mother and said, "Did you hear that?" Phil turned to a group of family and friends and announced, "Guess who's going to see a hooker next Friday."

Mike's jaw dropped. He swung his eyes to his father, and asked, "How'd you stand growing up with him?"

Steve laughed. "Learning to dodge him made me the most agile football player in Spartan history."

Clare pulled Mike's ear and said, "You're too young to see a hooker, baby. No man should see a hooker."

Phil told Mike, "Change your name to *Noman* and you'll have Nonna's permission to roam Hooker-Land."

Shooting Phil a dirty look, Clare turned to Mike, and said, "To think I actually encouraged him to talk when he was two."

"Uncle Phil's teasing, Nonna. She's a nice girl from C. A. Hooker College."

Before Mike turned to walk away, he pointed to his uncle, and said, "I'm forwarding all Nonna's sex-ed texts to you."

"Sex-ed never hurt anyone." He gave Steve a sideways glance. "Did you ever tell him how Mom caught us filling up condoms with—"

Steve held up his hand and asked, "Did you see Jenna?"

Pointing to the patio, Phil said, "Right there talking to her friend, Samantha."

"Great," he said. "She'll be on the phone for another hour."

Mike glanced in the direction of the French doors. "She's not on the phone, Dad."

Steve swung his eyes to the patio. "Sam's here?"

Mike said, "She walked in while you were playing bocce." Pointing to his uncle, he asked, "Who's wackier, Jenna's friend or him?"

Steve shrugged. "It's like choosing between a severe case of hemorrhoids or constant heartburn."

Ignoring his brother's insult, Phil nudged Mike. "Let's check out my competition."

"What do you have against The Friends of Jesus, Jen? They invite me to supper. They let me watch Lily."

Reaching for her drink, Jenna stretched out on the green and white striped chaise lounge, and said, "I never heard of that church, Sam." She sipped her drink and added, "I'll Google it tomorrow."

Sam stood, placed her hands on her hips, and shot back, "I'd rather you trust my judgment." With heated accusation, she added, "You nagged me to join a church. You told me to get to know some nice people. Well, I joined a church, and the people are nice. Now, you want to investigate them like they're criminals."

Heads turned toward Sam's high-pitched voice when she yelled, "You channel my mother more than anyone I know. What's wrong with all you people? Why do I constantly have to fight to convince you that I have a brain?"

Mike and Phil eyed Sam looming over Jenna. Jenna casually waved them to disregard the conversation. Turning to Sam, she said, "Sit down before you cause a scene."

"Stop treating me like a child," Sam countered with a voice reaching DEFCON 1. "You told me to join a church. I joined a church. That's not good enough for you." Shifting from one leg to the other, she swept the patio with her hot eyes. "Nothing's ever good enough for any of you."

Tension mounted, prompting Phil and Mike to move closer to the storm. Phil asked, "Refreshments anyone?"

Ignoring Phil, Sam crossed her arms over her chest and fixed her eyes on the guests cooling themselves in the pool.

Jenna stood and said, "We're fine."

Sam swung her eyes to Phil and blurted out, "I'd like some vodka."

Jenna gently shooed Phil and Mike away and touched Sam's elbow to direct her away from the crowd.

"When I said join a church, I was thinking more like the Catholic Church, the Lutherans, or the Baptists. Even a reputable synagogue or mosque."

Sam ripped her arm away and exploded. "You think a mosque filled with terrorists wrapped in turbans who lop people's heads off is better than The Friends of Jesus?"

Touching Sam's shoulder, Jenna said, "Shhh, not all Arabs are terrorists, Sam."

Sam stepped back and yelled, "Don't touch me, and don't shush me!"

Jenna raised both hands, palms facing Sam. In a softer voice, she said, "Even if The Friends of Jesus is a reputable organization, learn more about the parishioners before you share your life story. Don't make it easy for con artists to drain you out of your life savings."

In a cold, deliberate voice, Sam said, "You have an evil mind. I drove all this way to share good news, but you're not interested in celebrating my happiness. You'd rather celebrate another birthday for that brat who isn't even your kid." Her icy stare landed on Mike staring back at her from a few feet away. "I bet they lavish all kinds of money on you all year, and like a little fart, you don't even appreciate it."

"Stop, Samantha. He doesn't have to feel guilty for having people in his life who care about him."

Silence swept across the patio as guests discretely escaped indoors where word quickly spread of the confrontation near the pool. Steve reached the patio door just as Sam snatched a plastic fork from a glass table and yelled, "If I had a knife, I'd—"

Phil grabbed Sam's wrist and whispered close to her ear, "I'll take that."

Jenna stood in shock as Sam dropped the fork and glared at Phil.

Slipping his hands to Sam's shoulders, he gripped her, and said, "You don't want to hurt—"

Like a ferocious cat with its claws extended, Sam swiped close to Phil's face, and said, "Don't you ever touch me again!"

She raced across the lawn to her car. Blazoning with rage, she screamed back, "I don't need a birthday party. I don't need any of you." Her tires screeched as she sped up the quiet street.

Eyeing Jenna, Phil quipped, "Your friend's eleven eggs short of a dozen."

"Please, Phil. Not now."

More sympathetic, he said, "I need an honest answer. Was she drunk? If she's a danger to herself or other drivers, we have to notify authorities."

Staring toward the street, Jenna said, "She's sober now, but by tonight . . ." Her voice trailed off.

She turned to walk into the kitchen when Steve blocked her path. "Mark Packard warned that she could unravel."

She pushed past him in silence.

As she helped Jenna and Clare clean up the kitchen, Rosie wondered aloud. "How could I be at this party and not see Sam come or leave? Maybe all she needed was a hug."

"That girl needs more than a hug," Clare told Rosie as they joined their husbands on the patio. "Imagine if a mad dog would've marred her for life when she was three. The authorities would've put that dog to sleep the next day. Why do we give pedophiles so many chances?"

Tony added, "Follow the money. While we try to stop fathers from molesting their daughters, there's a thriving multi-billion dollar business in child trafficking across the world."

Rosie shook her head in disgust. "Look at the perpetrators. Often, they're the pillars of the community, doctors, lawyers, teachers, and preachers. They go on exotic vacations to South America or Asia to have easy access to children. So much evil!"

"Before we fall down a deep, dark hole of despair," Domenic warned, "I read somewhere that if you add up all the atrocities perpetrated by mankind since the dawn of creation, evil would be a small percentage compared to the good mankind has achieved over the millenniums."

"That's good to know, but somehow that fact doesn't strike me as consolation for children who cry at night after being molested by the people who are supposed to protect them," Rosie said with dismay.

In the kitchen, Jenna folded a dish towel, placed it on the counter, and turned to join her family on the patio, when her phone rang. Heavy breathing accompanied the sound of shattered glass in a sink.

"Sam?"

More heavy breathing.

"What broke, Samantha?"

Fumbling the phone receiver, Sam's muffled voice said, "My heart when I was . . . when I was . . . I think I was three. Or maybe . . . Maybe myknee when I was one, or was it my . . . my . . . my elbow? Yeah. Always somethin' breaking." A child-like voice shook when she asked, "Did you know mydaddyhurt me?"

"I can't understand what you're saying, Sam."

"How can you? How can anyone understand? So many people at that party. Theyall love you." Whimpering, she said, "Justwanted one. Only one person . . ." Her voice trailed off.

"I love you, Sam. You're like my sister."

"Oh yeah! Is that why you let your ugly FBI brother-in-law paw me like an animal in heat?"

"He thought you were going to stab me."

"Did I ever hurt you? Did I ever hurt anyone? No! So, how come everyone gets ta hurt me?" she whined.

"I'm tired of fighting, Sam. Just be careful not to cut yourself, okay?"

"Likeyoucare," Sam mumbled. Hurling more vitriol at Jenna, she said, "If you realy need to know, my empty bottle slipped. Slipped in the sink." Pitting Jenna against her new-found friends, she let out a sinister laugh and slurred her words saying, "The Friends of Jesus don't find if I rink. I mean mind if I drink." Her child-like voice rambled. "When I told . . . I told Sister Kelly fy mavorite color was purple, she bought me a bottle of wine. Put a purple bow on top. You never bought me diddly squat." After a slight pause, a guttural "Hmmm" sound rose from her before she reprimanded herself saying, "No parties for you. Not good enough. I know why, too. I know why." Unleashing her final accusations of the night, she said, "Can't stand me being happy. My mother told me over and over, you'd turn against me. Won't ever let me be happy." After a short pause, she whispered, "Guess what, Jenna. I'm smarter than the FBI, and I'm smarter than that psycho quack who murdered Josh. Oh yeah. I showed my mother." In between gulps, she said, "I realy love you, Jen, but, but, but not everyone else. They all, all of them deserve to die." There were more muffled sounds before the phone went dead.

Snapping her eyes shut for a second, Jenna looked up and caught Steve staring at her. Raising the phone above her head, she said, "The Friends of Jesus love her more than I do."

Pouring a glass of wine, Steve said, "Tell her Jesus is our friend, too."

Put off by his lack of sympathy, she said, "Don't poke fun at my friend's life spiraling out of control." Clutching the teardrop diamond hanging from her neck, she added, "Why's it so hard for you to understand that she needs help, not ridicule?" Turning her back to him, she dropped the phone on the counter.

He set his drink near the phone and said, "I worry about her, too, but I understand the difference between a helping hand and a lifetime of devotion."

Softening, she took a sip of his wine, and said, "Sam's angry, bossy, and even manipulative, but she's never been physically violent toward anyone. She was possessed out there."

"Does that surprise you? She demolished a church marquee and landed in a psych hospital. She uses you to re-enact vicious, verbal battles with her dead mother whom she hates." A wry smile crossed his lips. "Her threats make the anaconda between my legs cringe at the thought of being near her."

Fighting the urge to smile at the image he conjured, she said, "She's always ranted ad nauseam about her innocence, that she's the victim, but lately, she makes it a point to remind me how her mother gleaned her brilliance moments before she died."

He popped a cookie into his mouth and said between chews, "If for one moment you'd turn off the eternal fountain of sympathy you have for her, you might notice that she's been manipulating you with her sob stories for years. Face it, Jen, she may be incapable of differentiating fantasy from reality."

Jenna crossed her arms over her chest and admitted, "There's no mistaking the evil in her eyes when she threatened Phil. My blood curdled." Holding up the phone, she said, "The sound of her voice just now telling me her parents deserved to die chilled me to the bone." She stared past the French doors to where her own parents sat on the patio. Refusing to believe the worst of Sam, she turned to Steve, and said, "This is nonsense. It's her bitterness talking. I even believe her parents deserved to die." Letting out a light laugh, she concluded, "She's a maniac not a murderer."

He held his hand up palm facing her and proclaimed, "You're incapable of objectivity when it concerns Sam. Phil's convinced she's a sociopath and plans to review the evidence in that double murder. Mark Packard's holding back on Sam's self-defense claim, too. I don't know what that cop has on her, but it's enough to make him dog her for years."

Jenna leaned on the counter and drank from a bottle of water. "If Phil finds evidence, I'll change my mind, but not until then."

Steve grabbed her hand and pulled her toward the patio. "Maybe some fresh air will clear your head."

She surveyed the flower garden just beyond the pool. A light early evening breeze carried the fragrance of an overgrown lavender butterfly bush. The garden was comforting until she settled on a diseased sunflower, its head dried and drooping among several vibrant others of its kind lined along the fence. The petals shriveled at the edges; the flower's head hung threatening to break off with the slightest provocation. Unable to look away, she wondered if the dying flower cried a desperate, "Help," to the nearby white and pink asters blooming with hearty flair.

"How can Sam be surrounded by so much life yet only move through shadows and darkness?"

Following her eyes, he drew her close, and asked, "Did I ever tell you about the time I graduated from kindergarten, and Miss Betters gave each of us a two-inch pine to plant in our yards?"

Jenna shook her head.

"I was so excited about that sapling. I watered it faithfully and nagged my dad to fertilize it. Within a few years, that blue spruce grew to be the envy of the neighborhood."

"By now it's probably towering," she said, her eyes growing misty.

"We moved in July. The heat was so hot the Wicked Witch of the West would've melted in her own sweat. The old maid who bought the house wanted my tree out of her yard the week she moved in." His eyes held the dying sunflower in the garden. "Dad asked her to wait until fall so the tree would transition more easily, but she refused. He did his best to preserve the roots, but ..." He shook his head. "I was nine years old the spring when all the needles fell off. I hovered near my dad, watching him dig it out of the ground and chop up the branches. I helped pick up the twigs from the yard." He looked down at Jenna and said, "I still hate that lady."

Eyeing him with mild suspicion, she asked, "Did you really nurse a pine tree when you were five?"

Feigning insult, he raised his hand to heaven. "Honest! She forced my dad to dig a five-foot pine out of her yard on the hottest day of the summer."

A faint smile crossed her lips as she wondered aloud. "What if The Friends of Jesus doesn't even exist?"

"Packard warned us. He said she could be intellectually savvy, yet emotionally and morally stunted. Without sustainable roots . . ." Raising his brows, he said, "This ride's not over, Jenna."

Worry hung on Jenna like a heavy, oversized coat. After several moments of silence, she said, "You cried over a tree. What will I do if she—"

Before she completed her thought, Mike and his friends playfully pushed and shoved each other as they filed into the kitchen.

Steve motioned for them to stay inside as he and Jenna joined them.

Mike hugged his father, turned to Jenna, and said, "Thanks for the party. You always make coming home nice." Sheepishly eyeing her, he said, "I'm sorry if I upset your friend. I didn't mean to—"

Jenna held his face with both hands and said, "You were a gentleman, sweetie. I should've isolated her the moment she arrived."

Mike asked, "Was she on something?"

Rolling her eyes, Jenna said, "If we can get her on something, she'd think and act like a normal human being for a change."

Steve crossed his arms over his chest and said, "Let us worry about Sam." Motioning his head toward Clare and Tony, he said, "Tell them goodnight." Smiling, he added, "I'll be serving my *Almost Perfect Pancakes* for breakfast at nine sharp."

Mike gave his father a thumbs up and joined his grandparents.

Leaning back against the kitchen counter, Steve said with soft indictment, "You're a glutton for punishment."

Steely-eyed, Jenna countered, "When life hurts us, we retreat in love. When life hurts Sam, I'm her only poor excuse for respite."

He set his drink down and danced up close to her in sync with the music streaming through the kitchen speakers. Smiling at his sensuous hip bumps, her eyes swung to the patio then back to him.

"Our parents and those college guys are ogling us."

"Great! Let's show them life's a song we dance to, and love motivates every step."

Swinging a dish towel over her head and letting it soar to the table, she extended her hand. Taking hold, he twirled her around.

As Jenna and Steve glided across the kitchen, Mike tapped his grandmother's shoulder. "Look who's still partying, Nonna."

Clare called to Rosie, pointed, and said, "Let's pray their party never ends."

Chapter Twenty-Five

Weeks after Samantha's dramatic defense of The Friends of Jesus at Mike's birthday party, she began to fixate on another worry. Sam told Jenna, "Reverend Bill always keeps Lily tucked away in his office with the door closed." Mustering a level of conviction, she added, "I know he's hurting her."

"I keep telling you, Phil ran a check on Bill and Kelly Fitzgerald the day after you left the party. They came up clean."

"So, now you're on their side?"

"I'm telling you you're right," Jenna said, hoping to prevent a meltdown. "They're being good friends. If you want me to talk to them, I—"

"Oh sure. Like your mother talked to Child Protection Services when I was little? No thanks. I'll take care of him myself."

"Stop talking like Don Corleone, Sam. I swear you enjoy making people think you—"

After some heavy breathing, Sam yelled, "I didn't kill my mother!"

"I know you didn't kill her, but your loose talk causes people to wonder."

Sam's anger disintegrated into a whine. "I know I have a mean mouth, but everyone at Mike's party heard you warn me about Reverend Bill." Between soft sniffles she said, "I know he's bothering Lily. He even tried to get at me once, Jen, but I was afraid to tell you. You would've said, 'I told you so' like my rotten mother." After letting out a deep, long groan, she said, "I'm so sick of people hurting me."

"Reverend Bill isn't your father, and Lily isn't you. Give people a chance. Stop trying to outdraw people who you think are out to get—"

"I wish you'd stop telling me to stop doing this and stop doing that. People won't be happy until I stop breathing." After a short pause, Sam added, "He threatened to kill little Lily if I told on him." With frightening determination, she said, "She needs me."

"Why didn't you leave the church when Reverend Bill first bothered you?"

"Here we go with the interrogation." Reaching for her half empty bottle of wine, Sam told Jenna, "You're one of the main reasons why I drink."

Jenna countered, "That's an excuse I haven't heard before. Whatever the reason, your drinking prevents doctors from prescribing meds to help you cope with your depression."

"Oh, so now you're accusing me of using being tortured by my parents as an excuse to get bombed?"

"Use any excuse you want, Sam. Just don't start blaming me for getting drunk is all."

"Don't act all high and mighty, Jen. You're not immune to bad judgment." She gulped some wine straight from the bottle and asked, "Did it ever occur to you that you're the one who's screwed up? Don't you think it's crazy to buddy around with the guy who killed your little brother?" Oozing sarcasm, she lobbed more insults Jenna's way. "Everyone knows the reason why I drink, but maybe you need a psychiatrist to find out why you're not loyal to your dead brother."

Growing impatient with Sam's verbal abuse, Jenna said, "I fought Mark's initial assessment of you, but you're hell-bent on proving him and that detective right. You made me look like—"

"I don't care a raging hyena's red ass what that killer told you," Sam screamed. "All you ignorant anuses dropping degrees like diarrhea out of the wazoo keep trying to blame me for what happened in my life. None of it's my fault! For God's sake, I was a baby! I was in diapers when they started hurting me!" Between strenuous sobs she screamed, "What was I supposed to do, sprout wings and fly away?" Still sobbing, she blew her nose into a tissue, and said, "I swear that cop thinks he's Inigo Montoya, and I killed *his* father, the way he hunts me down! If little Inigo's so thirsty for revenge, why doesn't he hunt down Doctor Mark *The Murderer* Packard and make him pay for what he did? Everyone knows he killed Josh."

Jenna palmed her head as she listened to Sam sob herself out of mania. A short, silent spell passed when Jenna, sounding more conciliatory said, "I used to understand what you were telling me, Sam, but lately your stories don't make—"

"Lately?" How would you know anything about me lately? In a renewed tirade, she screamed, saying, "You're too busy letting that pig screw you anytime he wants. You think you're special?" In between mean, sinister laughs, she said, "Just because you accommodate that buffoon on a soft bed he bought in a big, pretty house he built, doesn't make you any better than all the other women men screw anytime and anywhere they want."

Saturated with fatigue and anger, Jenna said, "I love you, Sam, but love doesn't require me to allow your negativity to seep into my life and poison the good around me. I need a break from your constant madness."

Sam screeched, "Go ahead. Take a break from my madness! I'll just sit here by myself and fantasize what the hell a break from my madness might be like!"

The silence made Jenna sag with guilt.

Pushing the door shut to the dishwasher, she turned to Steve wrestling with Noce on the floor.

"I should've been more patient with Sam."

Noce growled and tugged as Steve pulled at her toy.

"Maybe I'll spend tomorrow with her. Take her to lunch. Shopping will take her mind off her misery for a while."

Allowing the dog to win the stand-off and meander to her bed, Steve's eyes followed Jenna as she turned to gather some wet dish towels for the laundry.

He stood, dusted off his pants, and said, "Detective Tanner told Phil he believes Sam's responsible for sending him bizarre notes over the past decade. Mark Packard had the same concern." He popped some nuts into his mouth and said between chews, "The perpetrator cuts out letters from magazines and pastes the word pig all over a white sheet of paper." Scratching his head, he said, "Gee, I wonder who's obsessive enough to keep that maniacal activity alive for a decade?"

Facing him, she said, "Cops attract all kinds of unsavory people, Stephen."

"But only one disparages Tanner every time she talks to you." Following Jenna onto the patio, he said, "I'd feel better if you invited her here."

Her eyes dropped to his groin.

Pointing at her, he said, "That's right! Never question the depth of my love for you."

Good-naturedly, Jenna told him, "Placing her near your larger than life display of manhood would cause a seismic meltdown of her multiple personalities." Holding up her phone, she said, "I'll tell her to expect me by noon."

More seriously he said, "She could be dangerous, Jen. She resents your good fortune. She's incapable of appreciating the love and loyalty you've lavished on her for years. Her needs are insatiable, and she's grown more unstable."

The dog, begging for attention, wandered up to Steve and sat at his feet. Stroking Noce's head and scratching her belly when she rolled over, he told Jenna, "Three reputable men believe she's suppressing evidence of her full involvement in her parents' deaths. Doesn't that raise a reasonable level of concern about engaging with her alone?"

Jenna jutted her chin. "She's miserable all the time, obnoxious most of the time, and a pain in the ass sometimes, but she's not a killer."

Chapter Twenty-Six

Sam grabbed Jenna's arm, pulled her into the house, and said, "Hurry! Don't let them see you."

Tripping across the threshold, Jenna asked, "Since when aren't you allowed to have visitors?"

"I don't want them to know you're on my side."

"There aren't any sides, Sam." Shaking her arm free, Jenna said, "I'm starved. Let's find a restaurant and do some shopping afterwards."

"No!" Sam said, pacing the kitchen floor. Her breathing was shallow and her words rapid. "You should've warned me you were coming."

"Didn't you get my message?"

Peeking through the slats of the closed blind, Sam swung around. "What message?" She quickly added, "Doesn't matter. I didn't get it. You have to go."

Jenna's mouth gaped. Avoiding a confrontation, she said calmly, "Now that I'm here, let's buddy around like we did when we were young and carefree."

Sam stopped. She picked up a dish towel, wrung it tightly in her hands, and asked, "When was I ever allowed to be carefree?"

Bewildered by Sam's behavior, Jenna slipped into a chair at the table. With premeditated exuberance, she said, "So, let's be carefree today."

Shaking her head like a tail attached to an over-excited dog, Sam repeated, "Not today! Not today! Not to—"

Jenna stood, grabbed Sam to steady her, and said, "Stop it! Tell me what's wrong. Let me help you."

Breaking free, Sam swung the dish towel and smacked Jenna on the upper arm. Firing back, she said, "I don't need your help! You ask too many questions, and you blame me for everything."

Mild trepidation caught hold of Jenna as she made another attempt to calm Sam.

"I'll leave if you want me to, but at least sit with me for a few moments while I psych myself for the long drive back home." With a sheepish smile she added, "I sure could use a cool glass of water."

As though she were battling Tourette's, Samantha rolled her eyes, flung open the cabinet door, and jerked her head back and forth to keep Jenna in her scope of vision. When she pushed hard on the handle to the faucet, the water burst out, filling the glass quickly, causing the water to spray onto the floor.

"Look what you made me do!" Sam screamed. Shoving the glass into Jenna's hand, she dropped to her knees and began to wipe the floor dry. Looking up, she said with contempt, "This is your fault! I don't have time to . . ." She ran to the sink, gritted her teeth, and with all her strength, wrung the towel dry. She threw her hands in the air and said, "Now, look at this sink!"

Jenna stood and said, "I made the mess; I'll clean it up."

Wild-eyed, Samantha ripped the half-filled glass from Jenna's hand and watched with desperation as more water splashed to the floor.

"Just go home!"

Jenna jumped back.

Rather than risk irritating Sam further, she dried her wet hands on her pant leg and asked, "Is it okay if I use your restroom before I start back?"

"Use it and go," Sam muttered as she sprayed a second coat of disinfectant on the already sterile sink.

Jenna closed the door to the powder room, leaned forward on the vanity, and stared into the mirror. Sucking in a deep breath, she held it for a second before exhaling slowly. What's she planning to do, Jenna wondered. If I show too much interest, she's liable to go ballistic.

Her eyes slowly surveyed the obsessively organized, pristine bathroom until they settled on a magazine rack. Several magazines lined up perfectly except for one conspicuous corner of a page that protruded. She carefully pulled the magazine out and noticed the cover had the capital letter *G* cut from the article title, "The Great Escape." She covered her mouth with her hand to stifle a gasp. As she leafed through the pages, a soft sigh of relief escaped her when no other letters appeared to be missing from the pages.

She took care to return the magazine to the rack, making sure all the edges were flush. The pounding on the door made Jenna jump.

"A herd of elephants empties its bowels faster than it's taking you!" Sam yelled.

Palming her chest to catch her breath and slow her racing heart, Jenna opened the door, winced, and said, "Cramps. They won't let up."

Sam walked Jenna to the back door. She was carrying an orange, see-through trash bag filled with paper she was eager to dump in the outdoor incinerator. Standing on the bottom porch step, she eyed Jenna carefully and was about to question her when Sam's phone rang. She dropped the bag on the walkway, sprinted up the stairs, and ran into the house.

Shaking her head in wonderment, Jenna stared at the bag. She owns the cleanest garbage on the planet, Jenna thought.

The longer she stared, the clearer several magazine images appeared through the plastic, revealing pages that were cut and ripped to shreds. Shooting a quick glance at the back door, Jenna pulled apart the draw string, snatched a magazine, and shoved it into her purse. No sooner had she retied the plastic drawstrings, she looked up and watched Sam slowly descend the stairs eyeing her with suspicion.

Sam lifted the bag and offered a stiff apology. "I'm sorry, but if you would've called . . ." Steadying her eyes on Jenna, she told her, "Next time talk to me before you show up."

Certain that her pounding heart was about to reveal her trespass, Jenna said, "You're right. I should've confirmed my visit. That was inconsiderate of me."

Samantha's brow rose. A bright smile lit up her face. She dropped the bag, threw up her arms, and said, "Hooray for me! Finally, I'm right."

She grabbed Jenna and gave her a tight hug. Swaying her back and forth with delight, she inadvertently knocked Jenna's purse to the ground.

Panic gripped Jenna as Sam reached with one hand for the phone and compact that emptied onto the concrete walkway and grabbed the bag with the other hand. Lifting the purse by its straps, she said, "God, Jen! Are you carrying Fort Knox in this thing?" Swinging it back and forth like a pendulum, she said, "I'd be a hunchback if that load was hanging from me all day."

Masking her fear with a fake laugh, Jenna slipped the strap on her shoulder and held it close to her side. "You're right again. You just talked me into buying a smaller purse on the way home."

Sam tugged at the strap and asked, "Can I have this one when you're done with it?"

Forcing a smile, Jenna said, "Of course. I'll bring it next time I come."

Once more she eyed Jenna with suspicion. Pulling a silver letter opener from her pocket, she began to tap it several times on her open hand.

"I know what you're up to, Jen."

Forcing back the fear rising in her, Jenna casually turned and walked slowly to the front of the house with Sam following close at her heels. Standing beside her car in the driveway, Jenna turned and said, "I enjoy spending time with you is all."

"Really? Then why haven't I seen you in months?" Slapping the letter opener harder on her hand, Sam said, "I used to like visitors. Not anymore. I get the feeling they're searching for hidden bodies." Continuing her hard stare, she said, "Admit it. You all think I'm a murderer, don't you?" Her cold, steely eyes penetrated Jenna before she yelled, "Well, I'm not!"

Feeling safer in full view of traffic, Jenna opened her car door, turned, and asked, "After all these years, why won't you trust me?"

Sam's eyes caught some distant point when she said, "Every person I've ever trusted hurt me. So many people. I can't even count how many . . ." Her voice trailed off. Swinging her eyes to Jenna, she exploded with anger. "How can I trust anyone when I couldn't even trust my own mother and father? I had to kill . . ." pausing to catch herself, "him, but everyone thinks I'm the horrible monster, guilty of the crime of the century." Her fire-red eyes glistened as her voice rose. "They're the guilty ones! Everyone who didn't help me. Every single one who knew and didn't help me is guilty!"

A twinge of guilt tugged at Jenna when she recalled her mother's failed attempt to intervene when Sam lived in their neighborhood. She placed her hand on her purse carrying the tattered magazine that condemned her as a traitor.

Offering consolation, Jenna said what she always resorted to saying. "I love you, Sam. If I thought you were a bad person, I would've stopped talking to you a long time ago. Maybe someday you'll realize how much you mean to me."

Jenna slipped into her car, breathed a deep sigh of relief, and headed home.

Plopping down on the couch next to Steve, Jenna covered her face with her hands, and asked, "How could I be so wrong about her?"

Holding her close, Steve said, "Sympathy's your Achilles' heel."

"What was I supposed to do, abandon her like everyone else?"

"While you stuck around to ease her pain, maybe you eased your over-active conscience, too."

"That's great! Now I'm a self-serving enabler."

"Before you start flogging yourself, consider that Sam may be more cunning than any of us realize. A detective, FBI agent, and one of the best psychiatrists in the country are grappling with her possible deception."

"My God, Steve. She's targeting a cop, a preacher, and me."

He turned down the volume to the game. "Until we have proof, it won't hurt to be cautious."

She pulled the magazine from her purse and tossed it in his lap.

Steve's jaw stiffened with each mutilated page he turned. Looking up, he asked, "Does she know you stole this?"

"Are you kidding? All the while she ranted about how she couldn't trust people, there I was gathering evidence against her." Closing her eyes, she said, "Some friend I turned out to be."

He slammed the magazine on the floor. "Assume she knows we suspect her."

Worry mixed with amusement when she asked, "Do you really believe she sits around and plots murders?"

"If it's all the same to you, I'd like to hear what Phil has to say."

Jenna sat up, let out a sarcastic laugh, and said, "Sam created a hit list." Counting on her fingers, she said, "I'm on the list; Reverend Bill, Kelly Fitzgerald, Mark, Detective Tanner." Wide-eyed she asked, "Did I miss anybody?" Shaking her head, she added, "Why not include you, Phil, Mike, and my mom and dad?"

Dialing Phil's number, Steve said, "She loves your mother."

"Oh yeah? Lately, she's been ranting about how my mom didn't push Child Protective Services harder."

Steve rolled his eyes. "I guess everyone associated with a sociopath could be in danger."

The Sunday services at The Friends of Jesus chapel wrapped up with the congregation singing an enthusiastic rendition of "The Battle Hymn of the Republic." Reverend Bill stood at the entrance and shook hands, accepting accolades for his fire and brimstone sermon titled, *I Am My Brother's Keeper*. Afterwards, there was a dinner in the community center to raise money for the local women's shelter.

Several ladies helped Kelly Fitzgerald clean up the kitchen while Reverend Bill said goodbye to the last well-wishers. Only minutes earlier, Sam grabbed hold of four-year-old Lily's hand, stealthily guided her through the side door, and inconspicuously walked the toddler to the car parked at the curb.

Lily looked up at Sam and asked, "Did Mommy bring my PJ's?"

"I bought brand new jammies for you. Mommy and Daddy have to take care of all the people, so I promised I'd take care of you."

"Mommy always buckles me in the seat. Can I kiss Mommy goodbye?" she asked with wide-eyed innocence.

"She's busy right now, Lily, so let's go get an ice cream cone and make some popcorn."

"Can I get the sprinkles?"

"We can get all the colored sprinkles we want," Sam told her as she sped away.

Kelly Fitzgerald was finishing up in the kitchen, when Reverend Bill said, "Grab Lily and let's get outta here. I'd like to catch what's left of the game."

Kelly shot him a puzzled look. "I thought she was with you."

He tossed his robe aside and called, "Lily, let's go!"

Fear gripped Kelly Fitzgerald as she ran through the center and called Lily's name several more times. The deafening silence of the hall filled them with panic. Reverend Fitzgerald grabbed his phone and dialed 9 1 1.

Chapter Twenty-Seven

FLASHING LIGHTS FROM SEVERAL PARKED PATROL CARS CAUSED curious passers-by to gather in front of the church hall. Inside, Kelly Fitzgerald told the police officer, "Lily would never walk off alone. Someone had to . . ." Choking up, she dabbed her wet cheeks with a dish towel and pleaded, "Please, find my baby," then dissolved into heavy sobs.

More resentful, Reverend Bill handed over a record of parishioners who belonged to The Friends of Jesus congregation for the last five years, and said, "Someone has our daughter while you're wasting time insinuating my wife and I let this happen. Ask over three hundred people where we were when Lily disappeared." He pulled out his handkerchief, dragged it across his brow, and yelled, "Find my daughter!"

Undaunted by Reverend Bill's indignation and anger, Detective Tanner continued to study the list. Eyebrows raised, he pointed to Samantha Kind's name, and asked, "How long have you known this parishioner?"

Reverend Bill shrugged. "Samantha's relatively new to our church family, but we've grown fond of her, and Lily loves her."

"Are you in the habit of allowing your child to be around people you don't know well?"

The reverend narrowed his eyes. "When we're in a pinch, she helps out. The lonely soul never says no to us. We invite her to supper now and then to show our appreciation."

Puzzled by the detective's interest in Sam, the reverend asked, "Surely, you don't believe she's capable of this kind of treachery? She's a God-send."

Detective Tanner looked over the rims of his glasses. "Fifteen years ago, your God-send blew a hole through her father's chest at point blank range. She claimed self-defense. So, if you have any inkling that she may be upset with you for any reason, now's the time to tell me about it."

Reverend Bill covered his face with his hands and let the silence swallow him.

Laughing and eating ice-cream together, Samantha and Lily were sitting Indian style on a plastic tarp sprawled across every inch of Sam's kitchen floor. Sam patiently guided Lily's pudgy hand holding the child safety scissors. She helped her cut out letters from magazines and paste them on a collage. Absorbed in song, they didn't hear Detective Tanner, several other uniformed police officers, and a medic gather at the front door.

Carrying a search warrant in his breast pocket, Detective Tanner pounded on the door three times, and yelled, "Police! Open up!"

Samantha swung her eyes to the door. In an instant, she grabbed Lily, ran to the hallway closet, and crouched behind the vacuum cleaner. Squeezing Lily tightly in her arms, she said, "I won't let him hurt you. No one's gonna hurt you ever again," she whispered.

Barely able to breathe, Lily cried, "Daddy's gonna be mad. I want my Mommy."

"We're mad at him. He's a bad, bad man, and we're not lettin' him touch us ever again."

When the police swung open the closet door, they tugged at Lily's arm to free her from Samantha's grip. Sam dove on Lily and cried, "He can't have her! He hurts her!"

To pry Lily from Samantha's arms, a medic shoved a syringe with diazepam into Sam's upper arm. Within seconds, Sam's body lay limp. She mumbled between groans, "HehurtsLily. Don't . . . Don'tlethimhurt . . . Never ever stopshurting."

Angered and befuddled by the Fitzgeralds' easy willingness to forgive Sam's brazen act, Detective Tanner faced the realization that authorities would have to release Sam from the hospital once the medication wore off. Unwilling to watch Sam skirt another criminal act of violence, he solicited Dr. Mark Packard's help in a last-ditch effort to hold her under some form of supervision until he could investigate the incident further.

"Since Samantha Kind is a former patient, is it possible to admit her in your facility for observation, at least for the time the law allows? Nothing's adding up in this case. Kind accuses the reverend of being a pedophile, yet these people don't bat an eye. They're calling it a misunderstanding." With an exasperating sigh, he said, "I don't buy it. I'm dealing with people who act like a carload of passengers on the Disorient Express. Help me find out what's happening here."

Mark Packard hedged. "Without the Fitzgerald testimony, you can't charge Kind with a crime and force a psychiatric evaluation. You need Jenna Gaone to convince Sam to commit in her best interest."

The detective laughed. "Kind's a brazen one-woman, delusional, vigilante committee. The Gaones know it, and you know it. Help me put this to rest before we end up with a body."

Mark Packard phoned Jenna and said, "Sam's in serious trouble. She kidnapped Lily Fitzgerald late this afternoon."

Jenna palmed her face. "Good God! I was with her around noon today. She was agitated and desperately wanted me out of her way. I should've never left her alone."

"The Fitzgeralds are letting it slide, but Detective Tanner has valid concerns. Tanner wants me to hold Sam at the Institute as long as I can to give him time to find out what's motivating the Fitzgeralds to be unnaturally complacent."

"Finally," Jenna said. "It's about time he's thinking straight." Her voice weighed down with guilt, she added, "I should've believed her, Mark. Mercy isn't motivating those people. Several weeks after she joined The Friends of Jesus, Sam began insisting that Reverend

Bill was hurting Lily. She obsessed on making him stop." Jenna sat down and held her head. "I treated what she was saying like it was just another one of her rants. There are times she goes on for months about an injustice, then," Jenna snapped her fingers, "like that, she drops it. She's never acted on any of them."

"Did she ever threaten to kill her father?"

"She always wished him dead, but she hated her mother more."

"How about if we hook up a phone conference with Detective Tanner? Be in his office at noon tomorrow so we can coordinate a plan. Whatever their reason, Samantha's fortunate the Fitzgeralds aren't pressing charges. Tanner's still adamant about not letting her walk. Admitting her to my facility may offer her an opportunity to gain some stability and give her leverage in a court of law if she should face future charges."

Jenna and Steve arrived at Detective Tanner's office earlier than expected and waited for Mark Packard to call. Rather than chance incriminating Samantha further, Jenna decided to stay mum on yesterday's encounter with Sam.

"This case grows more bizarre each time I turn around." Tanner tossed his glasses on the desk and narrowed his eyes. "I also find it interesting that you don't have much to say on the subject, Mrs. Gaone." Leaning back in his chair, he pointed at Jenna. "Your friend's unsavory, but so are this preacher and his wife, so do us all a favor and sign the papers to hold her in Packard's facility until I can figure things out."

"I can't sign papers if Sam's lucid, but Sam'll sign if I convince her it'll keep Lily safe."

Sitting back, he said, "Good. I'm all for keeping people safe." He tossed a folder onto his desk, shook his head, and asked, "What kind of people allow someone to terrorize their kid and don't make an issue of it? What kind of Christian doesn't think about the next poor kid Kind decides to snatch in one of her delusional episodes?"

Jenna shot Tanner a cold stare. "There won't be another kid unless that kid's being molested."

Wide-eyed, the detective asked, "Did you just confirm she's capable of doing this again?"

"For once, stop hearing only what you want to hear, and listen to what I'm saying. Don't allow your irrational pursuit of Sam to blind you. Reverend Bill isn't who he portrays himself to be, and neither were Sam's parents."

"And you know this how?"

"Sam was battered all her life. She perceives any child being hurt as an extension of herself. She's had plenty of opportunity to retaliate, but she hasn't. Did Lily seem traumatized when you rescued her?"

Tanner covered his face with his hands for several seconds before saying, "No, not in the least." Eying them, he said, "But make no mistake. Samantha Kind's a volcano. She's capable of lying dormant for years, but when she erupts, she takes a toll. Next time, we may not be so lucky."

Jenna softened. "No one's denying that Sam's troubled, but she's not a murderer, and she's not a kidnapper. If Sam took Lily, it's because she wanted to protect her."

The detective tapped his pen on the desk. "I have a feeling you knew Samantha Kind was planning to take this child all along."

"Don't say another word," Steve cautioned. "He's trying to make you an accessory to the crime."

Detective Tanner threw his hands in the air. "Give me a break, Gaone. Your friend blew her father away and maybe her mother, too. Then she kidnaps a preacher's child." He pointed to Jenna and said, "You're right. Instead of hiding the girl from us, she sat wide open on the kitchen floor singing and pasting collages about what they love most in the world." Shaking his head in frustration, he added, "Then, I have to figure out why this preacher acts like someone kidnapping his kid is like having his house toilet-papered by a group of sophomores after a high school football game." He swung his eyes to Jenna. "Side-stepping a molestation charge can explain a lot of unnatural behavior, excuse the pun."

Calmer, Steve said, "When Sam first started complaining about Reverend Bill, we let Sam know my brother, Phil, ran an FBI check on Fitzgerald. He came up clean."

Tapping his pen on the desk, the detective said, "I remember talking with Special Agent Gaone. Maybe it's time I give him another call." He shot Jenna a puzzled look. "What is it about this dysgenic lady that made you disregard your concern for the well-being of a child?"

"If I reported every threat-like rant Sam made over the years, they'd have to hire a *Sam-squad* just to handle her harmless verbal assaults." Jenna closed her tired eyes for a moment. Looking up, she said, "Despite the monsters who conceived and raised her with all the finesse of Attila the Hun, it's a miracle that Sam isn't a carrier of bad genes. If she were inherently evil, she would've carved out her father's heart as soon as she was old enough to wield a knife. It would've been so easy while he was in one of his drunken stupors."

Before Detective Tanner could counter, his phone rang.

"Dr. Packard, you're right on time. The Gaones are in my office. Let's straighten this mess out."

Over the next thirty minutes, they agreed on a plan to transfer Samantha Kind to The Art of Healing Institute. Sam would receive much needed help, and Tanner would have the time he needed to tie up the loose ends of the Fitzgerald kidnapping case.

Chapter Twenty-Eight

Samantha Kind forced herself to be a model patient at The Art of Healing Institute. Without liquor to dull the cruel reality of her mounting legal and emotional problems, she quickly slipped into a dark depression.

Nearly three weeks after the kidnapping incident, Reverend Bill Fitzgerald contacted Dr. Mark Packard to set up an appointment to visit Sam. He wanted her to know that The Friends of Jesus congregation was praying for her recovery, and it eagerly awaited her return to the fold.

Considering Sam's serious allegation against Reverend Bill, Dr. Packard found it curious that the reverend would willingly place himself in a perilous position with Sam so soon after her vehement accusation.

Hoping to flush out Reverend Bill's true motive for the visit, Dr. Packard hid his suspicion of the pastor and told him, "Your visit will do wonders for her recovery."

Unaware of Sam's plan to meet with Reverend Bill that same Saturday, Jenna drove to the Institute to spend the day with her and found Sam distraught at the prospect of meeting with Reverend Bill that late afternoon. Jenna sat across a cafeteria table and whispered, "Wouldn't it be grand if he incriminated himself?"

Sam pulled back. Anger rose in her when she asked, "You think that creep's dumb enough to admit what he does?" Eyes glistening, she stared across the cafeteria to a distant point. Under her breath, she said, "He deserves to die."

"No, Sam. He deserves to rot in jail for what he did. Think about it. If he wants to taunt you, wouldn't it be sweet if you captured his victory lap on tape?"

Sam's eyes swung to Jenna.

Jenna held up her phone. "Carry it in your pocket. Maybe he's arrogant enough to reveal something that will plant suspicion in Kelly Fitzgerald's mind." Her eyes grew large when she pointed at Sam and warned, "Don't dare breathe a word to Mark about our plan. He'll end it because it's probably illegal. If Bill incriminates himself, Phil will advise us what to do next."

Sam slipped Jenna's phone into her pocket and walked back to her room. Jenna left the Institute and drove to a nearby diner to wait for Sam's meeting with Reverend Bill to end.

Dr. Packard asked Reverend Bill to wait in his office while he coaxed an increasingly agitated Samantha Kind to meet with the preacher.

Twisting a tissue so tightly it shredded in her hands, Sam said, "No! Don't make me." Blinking back hot tears, she said, "He hurts Lily, and he'll hurt me." She punched her knee. "I promised Lily. Now, he has her, and she'll never trust anyone again." Through gritted teeth, she asked, "Why'd I have to be crazy?"

Dr. Packard pulled up a chair and sat across from her. "I share your uneasiness about the man, but you're the only one who can get him to drop some clues. If he's confrontational or threatening, we can give Detective Tanner a reason to follow up."

Gripping the phone in her pocket gave Sam a sense of urgency. "Okay, okay, I'll talk to him," she said, wiping her wet cheek. "Give me a couple of minutes. I don't want him to know I was crying."

After fiddling with the phone for a few seconds, she tucked it back into her pocket and gave it a secure pat. As she followed a nurse to the garden, Dr. Packard escorted Reverend Bill to the courtyard where Sam waited.

Dr. Packard exchanged pleasantries, walked to a nearby table, and reminded several nurses to keep a close eye on Sam. Returning to his office, he stood watch at a window that gave him a bird's eye view of the interaction between Sam and Reverend Bill.

As patients and their families mingled at surrounding tables, Reverend Bill sat across a patio table from Samantha and said softly, "You caused quite a stir. Lily doubts me now."

Samantha pierced him with a glacial stare.

Reverend Bill scanned the landscape for several seconds before resting on Sam.

"Did you know that in some New Guinea societies there are religious ceremonies that call for sexual contact between adults and children?" With a self-assured smile, he added, "Loving a child isn't frowned upon."

"Is that why you started a church? To get your filthy hands on kids' genitals and tell them they're not holy if they say no to you?"

"I can't believe Packard wastes all this money, time, and effort on misfits like you." Taunting her, he said, "Your parents must've been a helluva pathetic pair to spawn a degenerate like you. My Lily's special; she's my angel."

A nurse carrying a refreshment tray extended it to the reverend and Sam. Neither was interested.

A rare calm came over Sam when she told the reverend, "I'm glad Lily won't have to kill you."

A smug smile crossed his face. "You know nothing about my Lily."

He stood, buttoned his blazer, and arrogantly pulled at his cuffs. For aesthetic purposes, he leaned close to Sam, as if to offer a friendly kiss good-bye.

When Dr. Packard saw Sam push her chair back and jump up, he bolted to the courtyard.

Reverend Bill's venom-filled voice said, "Good riddance," as he slipped away seconds before Packard reached Sam's table.

Dr. Packard walked a visibly shaken Sam to her room where she sat in a chair, covered her face, and sobbed. Looking up with pleading eyes, she said, "Keep me locked up forever, but someone, anyone, has to stop him from hurting Lily."

"Did he say anything that would help Detective Tanner's investigation?"

Wiping her eyes, Sam said, "I want to talk to Jenna before I—"

Just then, Jenna popped her head into Sam's room and whispered, "How'd it go?"

Still shaken, Sam shoved the phone at Jenna, and said, "Take it. I don't ever want to hear his voice again."

His eyebrows raised, Mark Packard asked, "You taped him?"

Jumping to Sam's defense, Jenna told him, "I put her up to it. I didn't want you involved in case the plan backfired."

He eyed Sam and asked, "Did you get what you needed?"

Sam nodded.

As he turned to leave, he pointed at Jenna, and said, "I never heard this conversation."

Detective Tanner was listening to a dated radio interview between the comic Robin Williams and an NPR host when he bit into a chicken sandwich and forced spicy sauce to drip onto his pant-leg. He muttered an obscenity when he reached to answer the phone and a trail of sauce dripped onto his desk. Grabbing a paper towel, he wiped up the mess, and barked, "Detective Tanner, speaking."

"Phil Gaone, here. I have a recording of an incriminating exchange between Samantha Kind and Reverend Bill Fitzgerald."

Excitement seized him. "How'd the preacher get her to admit what she did?"

"On the contrary, detective. Fitzgerald's the one who makes a fart smell good."

Rolling up the paper towel into a tight ball, he tossed it hard across the room, and said, "You know we can't use that tape."

Phil laughed. "Just a minute ago you were dancing in the end zone at the thought of nailing Samantha Kind with it. Now that the reverend looks questionable, we can't use the tape?"

"We can't use it in court for either of them."

"I'm aware of the law," Phil asserted, "but the individual who passed the tape on to me thought the conversation might be useful to persuade Mrs. Fitzgerald that her husband more than likely is abusing their daughter. If she's not an accomplice, if she's not in denial, the tape might give her reason to schedule a physical with a pediatrician. Odds are slim that they'll find physical evidence of abuse, but maybe the doctor will pick up on the child's body language and verbal cues prompting a more thorough investigation into the interaction between father and daughter. Either way, Mrs. Fitzgerald can put the issue to rest; give herself peace of mind that she's protecting her daughter."

"Kind's so sure of Fitzgerald's guilt that she's willing to jeopardize herself?"

"The lady's on a mission to save the little girl."

"How soon can I get a copy of the tape?"

"I transferred the audio from a phone to an MP3. It's distinguishable enough. One favor."

"What's that?"

"As soon as Mrs. Fitzgerald hears the tape, erase it so the parties involved won't be threatened with law suits. Our common goal is to protect the girl. The tape's useless to us whether Mrs. Fitzgerald acts or fails to act on what she hears."

"Fair enough."

"I'll have the tape on your desk by morning."

Detective Tanner sat in an unmarked police car for over an hour waiting for Reverend Fitzgerald to leave his house for the community center. He knocked on the door knowing Kelly Fitzgerald was alone with Lily.

"May I help you?" Kelly Fitzgerald asked with apprehension.

"I have information about the incident involving your daughter that may interest you. May I come in?"

Masking her growing fear, she waved him in and motioned for him to sit. "Can I get you a cup of coffee?"

Shaking his head, Detective Tanner pulled a miniature recorder from his pocket, and said, "I've been trying to gather evidence on Samantha Kind for years, and she keeps slipping through my fingers. When you and your husband had every legal right to make sure we locked her up and threw away the key, your decision not to press charges baffled me."

"God calls us to act with mercy, detective. We know that Samantha's receiving the help she needs."

"That's a fact," he acknowledged. "Would you have been as quick to forgive Samantha Kind had Lily been harmed?"

She shot him an indignant, wide-eyed stare. "Had my baby been hurt, I still would've forgiven Samantha, but to protect other children, of course I'd want the law to handle it."

Eyeing her with sympathy for what she was about to hear, he said, "That's what I'm counting on. Listen to this exchange. What you choose to do after you hear it is your business. I won't bother you again unless you ask for my assistance."

Detective Tanner pressed *play* and watched Kelly Fitzgerald's face pale.

"Turn it off, "she whispered in a barely audible voice. "I heard enough." Crossing her arms over her chest, she locked herself in a tight hold.

Detective Tanner stopped the tape and just as quickly pressed erase. Walking toward the door, he stopped, turned to her, and said, "Do what you need to do to ensure your daughter's safety."

Between scrambling eggs and buttering the toast the next morning, Kelly Fitzgerald told her husband, "Lily has a doctor's appointment at one. I'll have to miss lunch at the community center."

Scanning the calendar on his phone, he said, "There's no appointment marked down."

"They called and asked if I'd fill a cancellation," Kelly lied, as she placed a plate of eggs on the table and poured him coffee. Diverting his attention, she asked, "You want me to pick up the dry-cleaning on the way home?"

"Yeah, do that." Brushing Lily's hair away from her mouth, he said, "It's a slow day today, so let me spend some quality time with my angel after the appointment. You can take the rest of the day off."

Turning her back to him to hide her anxiety, she dried some silverware, and said, "I just told you, Lily will be with me all afternoon."

Lily let out a cry when her father grabbed her face and planted a hard kiss on her mouth.

Kelly pulled her away from Reverend Bill and said, "Run upstairs and find your shoes. Maybe we can catch story hour at the library."

Wiping one eye then the other with her hands, Lily hurried up the stairs.

"What was that all about?" Reverend Bill asked.

"What do you expect from a four-year-old?"

Eyeing his wife with a lewd grin, he said, "Maybe she needs a little sister."

She shot him a glance then quickly looked away. Why not a brother, she thought. Oh God, I'm beginning to suspect his every word and action. What if he's innocent? I'm a regular Judas Iscariot, she thought, stealing a glance at the man she professed to love. She couldn't shake his sinister voice on the tape, his mean-spirited accusations toward Sam. With more resolve, she concluded, the man I believe he is would want me to protect Lily.

His hand on her shoulder made her jump.

"You're awfully edgy," he told her as he picked up his keys.

Catching her breath, she said, "Blame it on Adam and Eve. It's a monthly thing."

Grabbing his briefcase, he walked toward the door, turned, and said, "By the way, Lily was talking about a man who visited you." Puzzled, he asked, "What kind of talking machine did he show you?"

Her heart jumped to her throat. On the verge of being exposed for her cosmic treason, she began to fumble a story, when Lily burst into the room, tugged at her mother's pant leg, and whined, "Tie my shoes, Mommy."

Lifting Lily in her arms, Kelly breathed a sigh of relief for the interruption. She sat her on the edge of the countertop and slowly talked her way through the steps of how to tie a shoelace.

Pressed for time, Reverend Bill said, "I have to run. Be careful who you invite into the house, Kelly. We've been attracting some fruitcakes lately, and it's not even Christmas."

The doctor completed Lily's regular examination before she broached the topic of examining Lily's private area.

Lily shook her head and whined, "I wanna go home."

Holding her tightly, Kelly whispered, "Sometimes girls itch down there. Can the doctor see if you have a rash? She can make it better."

Lily clung harder to Kelly's neck and blurted out innocently, "I don't like it." Burying her face into Kelly's chest, her muffled voice said, "Sam told me no one's sposed to touch . . . No touching down there." More assertive, she looked at her mother and cried, "Not even mommy and daddies!" Burying her face again, she cried, "I don't wanna new mommy."

"I'll always be your mommy, and you'll always be my baby."

Lily pressed her knees together so hard, her tiny body quivered.

Rage mixed with fear and shame when Kelly said, "How could I not know?" Holding Lily tighter, she asked the doctor, "What do I do? How can I protect my child?"

A quick, preliminary examination confirmed abnormal activity. Calming Lily first by letting her play with a baby doll, the doctor casually asked questions to assess the extent of the abuse. With her mother at arms' length, Lily babbled about her father's trespasses and how he frightened her with removal from their home if she told anyone their special secret.

Lily wagged her index finger in the doll's face and said, "Nevvver, evvver tell. Your mommy won't like you anymore." She turned her eyes to Kelly and asked, "Are you mad at me, Mommy?"

Kelly gathered Lily into her arms and assured her. "I'll always love you to the moon and back."

The doctor escorted Kelly and Lily to her office where they called Detective Tanner and an advocate from Child Protective Services to advise them of her findings.

Chapter Twenty-Nine

SAMANTHA KIND SAT IN A CHAIR GAZING OUT HER WINDOW. She watched people tossing coins into the fountain situated in the center of The Art of Healing Institute's serene garden. "A silly, wasteful tradition," her mother drilled into her on more than one occasion. Still, she wondered how many of the wishes and dreams came true. A knock at the door startled her.

"You have a visitor," Dr. Packard told her.

Shrugging, she turned toward the fountain again, and said, "I don't feel much like talking."

"What if I told you Lily's safe, and Bill Fitzgerald won't be able to hurt her or anyone else for a really long time?"

Sam swung her eyes to Dr. Packard. "Lily's safe?"

He pulled up a chair and straddled it. "You kept her safe, and Jenna's here to make sure you're safe." Letting out a laugh, he said, "You have one heck of a helicopter friend."

Mist blurred Sam's eyes. Her lips trembled slightly when she said, "I've never been a good friend to her. She deserves a friend who tells the truth."

"You could've checked out weeks ago, but you stayed. Frankly, your progress astounds me. If you keep up this pace, I see a future where you'll be a better friend to yourself and Jenna."

Fixing her eyes on the fountain, she told him, "I used everyone, but I shouldn't have used Jenna."

"Sometimes we need to use people. We use them to get through the day. We use them to get stronger. When we're strong enough, we can let people use us."

Continuing her stare out the window, she said, "I'd like some ice water, please."

"I'll get that for you right now."

He left her room, but quietly pressed his back up against the wall outside her door for several moments. He hoped to catch another one of her routine, scathing monologues chastising herself.

Samantha didn't disappoint. Her voice carried shock, as though she just committed the deed. She scolded herself saying, "You can't tell her you killed them! She'll stop loving you." With disbelief in her voice, she said, "You shot them. She believes you had to kill them. You could've walked away." She cried out, "Why didn't you walk—"

"For you," Dr. Packard said, handing Sam the water.

Fear gripped her. Refusing the water, she followed him as he moved across the room where he placed the glass on a chest of drawers.

Weighed down by a life of pretense, her shoulders sagged. "No one believed me anyway."

"I believe people who should've loved and protected you victimized you. I believe you edited your memories to make life the way you wanted it to be, the way you needed it to be to survive. I believe you're tired, and you want to heal."

Nervously picking at her pant leg, she sighed. "What's the use? That crazy cop's gonna finally get to do his happy dance."

"Not necessarily."

Choking up, she admitted, "I killed them. There was so much blood." Her body shivered when she explained, "I scrubbed and scrubbed and scrubbed, but still," she whispered, "sometimes I still can see and smell all the blood."

"Why that night, Sam?"

Shrugging, she said, "I didn't plan it, but in a way, I planned it all my life." Her voice carried a hint of disbelief when she said, "I wanted to kill myself, but my mother stood there laughing." Mimicking her mother, Sam said, "She pointed her finger at her head and kept pretending to pull the trigger over and over and over again." Sam's fingers played with a string hanging from her sweater. "I begged and begged her. Please love me, Mommy, but she kept on . . . Why didn't she love me?" Sam whined. "I tried to hit her with the gun, but she reached out and grabbed my hand, and the gun went off, and she was dead." She sucked in a sob and said, "And I was glad she was dead."

"Where was your father?"

"He ran in when he heard the shot. He lunged at me." She locked eyes with Dr. Packard and stuttered, "I . . . I . . . I had to shoot him. He would've killed me." A haunted look possessed her when she held her head between both hands and pressed hard. "They're always here. They won't leave me alone," she said sobbing.

Dr. Packard handed her the glass of water and said, "Now that we can have an honest discussion, in time, we'll be able to put the ghosts to rest." His hand on the door knob, he turned, and said, "Right now, your best friend's waiting to see you. I suspect you'll have a lot to talk about."

His caring voice calmed her. Before he left the room, she said, "I thought you'd hate me."

Offering a warm smile, he said, "A wise man taught me that every worthwhile person has some sad stories to tell." He raised his brows and said, "Let's make a deal. I'll help you quail the demons; you help me be a better doctor."

A month later Sam sat near one of the flower gardens at The Art of Healing Institute and explained to Jenna how she experienced another milestone in therapy.

"At first I cringed at the sight of the massage therapist who rubbed my shoulders every day for one lousy thirty seconds." Comically rolling her eyes, she said, "We're up to one and a half minutes." Proud of herself, she said, "Sometimes the nurse leaves the room." She was quick to add, "But I make them keep the door open."

Just as Jenna high-fived Sam, Steve and Lily paraded down the path carrying a birthday cake aglow with candles.

"Surprise!" a chorus of friends sang out.

Lily climbed onto Sam's lap as the Rossi and Gaone families and friends sang *Happy Birthday* to Sam.

Overwhelmed by the attention, Sam buried her face in Lily's hair, blinked back tears of joy, and whispered, "Did you tell them it was my birthday?"

Lily pointed to Steve and said, "He invited me and Mom to the party." Lily caressed Sam's cheek and parroted what she heard the grownups discussing on the trip to the Institute: "From now on, we're all gonna help keep water out the ship."

"Close enough," Steve said, winking at Lily.

Mark Packard tapped a spoon on a glass to draw everyone's attention. He raised his glass and locked eyes with Dominic Rossi hugging Rosie.

"To people with hearts full of friendship and forgiveness, allowing us to grow in confidence and love." Before he excused himself for another appointment, he bent down and whispered to Sam. "If you need me when you talk to Jenna I—"

"I want to do this on my own," Sam insisted.

Eyeing her name on an envelope Sam clutched in her hand, Jenna nudged Sam, and teased, "You gonna give that to me in our lifetime?"

"It might be fifteen years too late."

A puzzled look crossed Jenna's face.

As friends mingled and doled out party food, Sam gently nudged Jenna back, and said, "Walk with me down to the fountain." Waving the envelope, she told Jenna, "You can read it there."

As they walked down the path together, Jenna stopped short of the fountain, grabbed Sam's hand, and placed it on her swollen belly until the baby ended its contortion act.

Sam smiled and said, "I'd give anything in the world to be in there instead of out here." Handing Jenna the envelope, she added, "You kept me alive when . . ." Her words stuck in her throat.

Tapping the envelope on her open hand, Jenna asked, "Aren't you a bit dramatic?"

"It's the truth."

Jenna opened the envelope and read Sam's lengthy apology for clinging to Jenna as though she were the only life raft in Sam's sea of despair. When Sam explained the truth of the day she killed her parents, Jenna swung her eyes to Sam and said, "I've always known the truth. They robbed you of who you were supposed to be. Truth?" she asked with disdain. "We should've done more. Something! Anything!" Filled with remorse, she stared at the fountain as the baby growing in her gave her a swift kick.

Letting go of her usual hostility, Sam offered a rare sober assessment of humanity. "People are so afraid to admit they're so afraid. Being around people like me scares them. Hell, it scares me to be me. They think if they get too close, my miserable life might rub off on them." Shrugging, she said, "Who knows? Maybe my misery reminds them of their own dance with the devil. That's what some people in our group sessions say about their family and friends." Letting out a sigh, she said, "I guess the world batters all of us, but some people are lucky enough to have someone or something that makes the battering worth enduring."

"Can you find what you need to make all the battering and bruises worthwhile?"

"I'm getting there, but life shouldn't be this hard. We're always struggling to make people like us, always fighting to be what the world wants us to be. We're so wrapped up in survival." She looked toward the gathering and said, "I'm surrounded by people who say they love me, but you're the only one who never let go of my hand. You never walked away." Her eyes watered when she stared at Jenna's round belly and offered a warning. "Don't ever let anyone hurt your . . . Never let go of your little girl's hand."

Fighting the mist in her own eyes, Jenna surveyed the rolling hills in the distance. She remembered when she did let go of her little girl's hand, and a part of her died. Standing with Sam in this garden, she felt reborn; their lives full of promise.

Turning to Sam, she said, "You saved Lily's life, and your phone calls that year I lived in France saved my life, too."

Not sure of Jenna's reaction, Sam asked, "Can a person be a life saver and still think about wanting to die?"

Trying hard to mask her concern at the revelation of Sam's resurgent sadness, Jenna said, "We all think about dying, Sam, but life gives us a chance to live a million moments helping each other learn, laugh, and love before we leave this earth."

Samantha locked eyes with Jenna. "Right now, this moment, I feel more love than I've felt my whole life," her voice cracked, "but all this affection scares me almost as much as the rejection."

Jenna extended her hand, and Sam grabbed hold. Wiping her cheek with her free hand and playfully tugging at Jenna, Sam asked, "Do you believe the more pain you feel, the more you can appreciate happiness?"

"That would make us the Wall Street of happiness, and you the prime investor," Jenna said, playfully.

As they walked hand in hand closer to where Steve stood with the other guests, a gray cloud overhead crept in front of the sun casting a shadow that brought on an extended chill.

Sam stopped Jenna and asked with child-like wonder, "How come you always answer the phone?"

As though it were a universal truth, Jenna assured her, "Love always answers."

Chapter Thirty

NOCE PLAYFULLY TUGGED AT HER BRAIDED ROPE TOY UNTIL a sharp pain stabbed Jenna in the side. Jenna let go and drew in a deep breath. Contractions crawled across her stomach several minutes apart. Waddling onto the patio, she told Steve, "It's time to go."

Dropping the book he was reading, Steve grabbed his keys and drove her to the emergency room.

A short hour later, six-pound, twelve-ounce Clara Rose Gaone sprawled across Jenna's chest, her tiny mouth searching for a protruding nipple. Steve basked in the love of his wife and child for only a moment before the recollection of Mike's birth washed over him, carrying with it waves of guilt. Ashamed that he had reacted with little interest in being a father back then, he wondered how Mike regarded the birth of his sister, the excitement that surrounded her arrival.

Jenna interrupted Steve's feeling of dereliction to say, "Her huge eyes are glued to my face the same way Carly stared at me." Looking up, she said, "I'll never let her go." Curling the fine strands of the baby's hair around her index finger, she asked, "Does Mike know he has a sister?"

"I called him a little while ago." Forcing a chuckle, Steve told her, "He asked if she's as good looking as he is. I told him she's prettier than all of us."

Catching his eyes before they fell, she said, "We both made mistakes with our first, but that didn't stop them from growing into good people. Because of them, we'll do better with Clara Rose."

Her words caught his heavy heart like a perfect wind catches a faltering kite, lifting it high, enabling it to soar.

The next morning, Steve walked into Jenna's maternity room hiding his face behind a spray of red roses. Before he could bend over to kiss her, Jenna's cell phone rang.

"I wonder why Mark Packard's calling so early."

Shoulders slumping, Steve placed the roses in a vase, and said, "This can't be good."

"Jenna, Sam's gone."

A frown quickly replaced her smile. "Gone? I talked to her yesterday and told her about my baby. She was excited. We made plans to bring Clara Rose for a visit in a few weeks. Why would she just up and—"

"You had your baby? I didn't know. Congratulations!" After a slight pause, he said, "That may explain why she signed release papers early this morning. I saw it coming, but I hoped I could head it off. News of your baby could've triggered memories of what she missed from her own mother, and it's a stark reminder that she'll likely never bear her own child."

"I'll talk to her, Mark. She'll be back. The Institute transformed her into a new person."

"No, Jen." His voice was sympathetic but firm. "She needs to come back on her own. Give her space. Let go of this burden for a while and enjoy your little girl. It's not easy to admit, but sometimes we can't help a person latch on to a healing memory, a reason to make life worth living. Sam's put up a helluva good front longer than any of us could fathom, but she's blocked off every artery through which friendship and love flow except for you. The best you can do for her now is keep listening. We'll talk next week when you're settled."

Shaken by Mark's call, she drew the baby closer and began to rationalize. "Sam talks about the lessons she learned in group therapy." With a tentative side-glance, she told Steve, "Maybe she learned to manage the anger and sadness better than we think." More to convince herself, she added, "Months of sobriety and intense therapy have to count for something."

A nurse knocked on the door to ask if the baby needed a diaper change. Shaking their heads in unison, she chuckled, handed Steve a diaper, and said, "Just in case the situation changes in the next few minutes."

The room was quiet again except for occasional soft voices travelling though the hallway.

Soon after the baby's noon feeding, Jenna was readying herself to say goodbye to Steve when her phone rang. All hope of Samantha being able to manage her pain slipped away when Jenna heard her garble, "Why'dthey hurtme, Jen? I was always a good liiittle girl. Help me. Help me be happy. I need . . . I need . . . I want my mom. I want my mommy ta . . . ta . . . ta hold me. You holdin' yer baby?" she asked between sobs. "It's gonna be okay," she whispered. "I'll be okay. It's gonna be okay, isn't it, Jen? My mom told me over and over and over, 'You can't trust anyone. Don't . . . don't . . . don't . . .' And I don't! Even Joshy wouldn't share his angel hair pasta with me," she whimpered. Make me angel hair pasta, Jen.

"Josh?" Jenna asked, surprised. "He used to sneak pasta to you every Sunday."

"Little Joshy. Every Sunday. Put it on my back porch. Last night, he kept pullin' it away. He looked so happy. I wanna be happy, too." At the end of a long, loud burp, she said, "Tell Josh ta share, Jen. He'll listen to you. Tell him fer me."

Goosebumps formed on Jenna's arms. The baby startled when her mother's louder than intended voice said, "Oh my gosh, Sam! My grandmother warned us never to eat with the dead in our dreams because if we ate with dead people, we'd have to stay with them. Josh and I were petrified to fall asleep for a week after she told us that story." Moving the baby to her shoulder, Jenna said, "Don't you see? Josh loves you so much; he's protecting you. He wants you to live. We want you to live."

A moment of sobriety came over Sam prompting her to ask, "Did yer grandma escape from some asylum or something? Sounds like something my crazy grandmother would tell me, if I had a crazy grandmother, which I don't. What kind of battle-ax tells a kid not ta eat with dead people?" After chugging more vodka, intoxicated madness returned when she garbled, "Ask any proctolo . . . proc . . . Whatever they call those asshole doctors, and he'll tell ya. It's probably safer ta eat with dead assholes. Alls living assholes do is betray and hurt you. Whocares anyway? Alls I wanted was some angel hair . . . Someone ta care 'bout me." With authority, she warned, "Don't let him touch her! Don't ever let him near her." She whispered, "Fathers hurt little tiny girls."

The familiar sound of a bottle clinking against glass turned Jenna's stomach.

Steve reached for the baby, but Jenna shook her head and drew Clara Rose closer.

When Sam abruptly ended the call, Jenna slammed the phone on the bed and cried, "What went wrong?"

"You mean besides two sadomasochists gutting the spirit out of their innocent kid?"

Anger rose in her as she cradled the baby in her arms. "Why did they give birth to a beautiful baby then turn around and abort every chance for her to have a good life?"

They both knew that question would never generate an adequate answer.

Sitting on the edge of the bed, Steve thought about how Jenna always rose like dawn in Sam's world of sunsets, how she constantly provided a flow of reasons for Sam to hold on and fight for one more day. He wished that help for abused children like the *Carly McCoy Foundation* provided would have existed when Sam was in grade school. Maybe Sam could have learned to fight the demons better.

The ring tone on Jenna's phone caught them by surprise.

Relieved, she told Steve, "It's Sam."

Between strangled sobs, Sam said, "Don't . . . Don't let him touch the baby." Falling to a whisper, she warned, "He'll hurt her, Jen." Louder, she said, "He'll hurt and hurt and hurt her. Won't ever go away. Even when they die. Even if you kill 'em. They still hurt and hurt and hurt us." Barely audible, she said, "It's so hard." After several sniffles, she said, "It hurts when I breathe, Jen. If I stop breathing, will it stop hurting?"

Again, Steve extended his hands for the baby, but Jenna shook her head hard.

Hurt by her ambivalence, he searched her face until the words Jenna's father used to describe the prominence she played in his life rolled off his tongue. "*Questa ragazza è il mio battito cardiaco.*"

Startled back to reason, her eyes apologetically signaled him to take the baby.

She told Sam, "I'm so sorry your father hurt you. Every child deserves parents who hold him or her like they're holding their own beating heart in their hands."

Steve retreated to a corner chair and tenderly brushed his cheek close to the baby's lips. Her soft, sweet breath renewed him as he listened to Jenna breathe hope into Sam's tortured soul.

After all the life that happened to them, they came around to where they first began, Jenna convincing Sam that "No one really lives a happily ever after in this world. Some people manage to keep the water out of the ship better than others is all."

"Been bailin' all my life, Jen. Tired of tryin' to clean up my filthy life. I clean and clean and clean. Won't ever come clean. Always drownin'. Water's always gettin' in. May's well stop breathing. Breathing hurts so much. You have a little baby to love you and . . . and . . . and . . . Her world's beginning. Mine's ending." She sniffled several times before bursting into uncontrollable sobs.

Playfully scolding her, Jenna said, "For God's sake, Sam. You sound like Chicken Little. The world's not going anywhere. California has three more hours, and some parts of the world like China are already living tomorrow."

Amid her sobs, Sam broke into loud laughter. "Problem solved! Movin' ta China. Nobody'll know me. Start all over again." She blew her nose and mumbled, "Problem is I know me." After a short silence, she said, "I'm so scared. Make me believe I'll be," she whispered a desperate, "okay."

Just then, Jenna caught Steve waltzing with Clara Rose to music only he and the baby could hear. Shooting Jenna a wink, he mouthed, "I love you."

Inspired by the warmth of him, she said, "We're all afraid, Sam. I was afraid to let myself fall in love, but because I took a chance, today I'm watching Steve dance with our baby. You were afraid to get sober, but because you did, Lily's safe. We can't let fear of losing and hurting trap us in a dream world. Life's never perfect like our dreams. Reality is stormy and messy, but it has music, mud pies, rainbows, and sunrises to lift our spirits and fill us with hope."

"I love rainbows, Jen, but I'm so tired. I wanna sleep. I wanna eat angel hair pasta with Josh."

"No, Sam! Josh said, 'Not yet.'"

"Joshy's dead, and I'm gonna . . . I'm gonna . . ." The phone slipped out of Sam's hand and disconnected Jenna.

Jenna pushed her head back on the pillow and focused her hard stare at the ceiling.

Steve slid onto the edge of the bed and said, "Someone's searching for food."

He watched Jenna guide the baby's mouth to her burgeoning breast. Tiny lips grabbed hold, and within seconds the over-sized nipple vanished into the baby's mouth, pumping rhythmically with soft ferocity. Steve looked on with wonder and asked, "Does that hurt?"

Relief set in as the baby emptied Jenna's gorged breast. "The more she eats, the less pain I feel." Continuing to fake calm, Jenna said, "Sam's spiraling out of control. What if I can't convince her this time, if I come up empty?"

He ran his index finger over her shiny, hard breast and teased, "That doesn't appear to be an immediate concern."

His tender touch felt like the healing hand of God coaxing her to relax long enough to muse, "I can't believe my boob's bigger than this baby's head."

Surveying her face, Steve wondered how much longer Jenna would be able to dispel the shadows looming over Sam's life. At first, he fancied her caught up in the vanity of being Sam's savior, but fifteen years was a long time to play guardian to a wounded person snared in pain and sorrow. He imagined Jenna's heart battling her head, convincing her that Sam would call again. Each time Jenna came to the precipice of despair over Sam, she'd flex her hardy spirit and rail against the world that turned its head, distanced itself, remained indifferent to Sam's pain and the cry for help from a million other battered children who people easily dismissed. Even when he balked, Jenna refused to let him lose sight of the fact that Sam and others like her were the victims. Not her. Not him. Not the world.

Steve knew Jenna had come to grips with the world's injustice that difficult day in France when she let go of Carly. The nuanced way she was tending to Clara Rose strengthened his certainty that she would rock the world before she let go of the baby or Sam. Grateful that Jenna never allowed the sad songs that surrounded them stop her from dancing to the sweet melodies that played in their hearts, he resolved to reciprocate the best way he knew how. He didn't know when the struggle to save Sam would end. He only knew that destiny married him to a heart so wide, and that meant he owned a share in the victory or defeat.

Acknowledgments

Thank you to family and friends who helped me on this artistic journey. Their advice and editing skills made the story better than it would have been without their creative and professional input.

David Antognoli---retired English teacher

Jason Antognoli----Emmy Award winning producer of a daytime series and script writer

Elaine Hoffman----retired librarian

Father James Downs---retired Catholic priest

Anne Koszela-------an avid reader

Myra Gabriel Cook----retired elementary teacher

Jan Wilson----------former State Police Officer and current Child's Protective Service coordinator

Kim Campbell-----current child psychologist

Teddi Black---Cover design

Megan McCullough---text layout

About the Author

Ann Abraham Antognoli was born and raised in New Castle, Pennsylvania. The sixth child of Lebanese parents, she learned to love *story-telling* as a child because her parents always told stories to teach life lessons. She earned a Bachelor of Science Degree in English from Edinboro University of Pennsylvania and a Master's Degree in English from Westminster College in New Wilmington, Pennsylvania. She taught high school English for over twenty-five years and lives with her husband David in New Castle, Pennsylvania. She and her husband are the parents of Jason, Erin, and son-in-law, Andy Cleavenger.

Other novels by Ann Abraham Antognoli: *The Sunny Spaces*

Made in the USA
Monee, IL
05 November 2026

67377187R00173